Advances in Patient Education: An Integrated Approach

Editors

LUCY W. KIBE
GERALD KAYINGO

PHYSICIAN ASSISTANT CLINICS

www.physicianassistant.theclinics.com

Consulting Editors
KIM ZUBER
JANE S. DAVIS

October 2024 • Volume 9 • Number 4

ELSEVIER

1600 John F. Kennedy Boulevard • Suite 1800 • Philadelphia, Pennsylvania, 19103-2899

http://www.theclinics.com

PHYSICIAN ASSISTANT CLINICS Volume 9, Number 4
October 2024 ISSN 2405-7991, ISBN-13: 978-0-443-24638-8

Editor: Taylor Hayes
Developmental Editor: Anirban Mukherjee

Physician Assistant Clinics (ISSN: 2405–7991) is published quarterly by Elsevier Inc., 360 Park Avenue South, New York, NY 10010-1710. Months of issue are January, April, July, and October. Periodicals postage paid at New York, NY and additional mailing offices. Subscription prices are $155.00 per year (US individuals), $100.00 (US students), $150.00 (Canadian individuals), $100.00 (Canadian students), $150.00 (international individuals), and $100.00 (international students). For institutional access pricing please contact Customer Service via the contact information below. Foreign air speed delivery is included in all *Clinics* subscription prices. All prices are subject to change without notice. Orders, claims, and journal inquiries: Please visit our Support Hub page https://service.elsevier.com for assistance.

Reprints. For copies of 100 or more, of articles in this publication, please contact the Commercial Reprints Department, Elsevier Inc., 360 Park Avenue South, New York, NY 10010-1710. Tel. 212-633-3874; Fax: 212-633-3820; E-mail: reprints@elsevier.com.

Physician Assistant Clinics is covered in *EMBASE/Excerpta Medica and ESCI*.

JOURNAL TITLE: *Physician Assistant Clinics*

ISSUE: 9.4

PROGRAM OBJECTIVE
The goal of the *Physician Assistant Clinics* is to keep practicing physician assistants up to date with current clinical practice by providing timely articles reviewing the state of the art in patient care.

TARGET AUDIENCE
Physician Assistants and other healthcare professionals

LEARNING OBJECTIVES
Upon completion of this activity, participants will be able to:
1. Review preventative medicines impact towards the prevention of disease and managing the welfare of health within communities.
2. Discuss the role of technology in patient education.
3. Recognize the urgent need for collaborative efforts among healthcare professionals, policymakers, and communities to dismantle structural barriers.

ACCREDITATION
The Elsevier Office of Continuing Medical Education (EOCME) is accredited by the Accreditation Council for Continuing Medical Education (ACCME) to provide continuing medical education for physicians.

The EOCME designates this journal-based CME activity for a maximum of 16 *AMA PRA Category 1 Credit*(s)™. Participants should claim only the credit commensurate with the extent of their participation in the activity.

All other health care professionals requesting continuing education credit for this enduring material will be issued a certificate of participation.

DISCLOSURE OF RELEVANT FINANCIAL RELATIONSHIPS
The EOCME evaluates the relevancy of financial relationships with its instructors, faculty, planners, and other individuals who are in a position to control the content of CME activities. The EOCME will review all identified disclosures and mitigate financial relationships with ineligible companies, as applicable. An ineligible company is any entity whose primary business is producing, marketing, selling, re-selling, or distributing healthcare products used by or on patients. For specific examples of ineligible companies visit accme.org/standards. EOCME is committed to providing its learners with CME activities that promote improvements or quality in healthcare and not a specific proprietary business or a commercial interest.

The authors and editors listed below have identified no financial relationships or relationships to products or devices they have with ineligible companies related to the content of this CME activity:
Edward Adinkrah, MD, MPH; Felix Alvelo, MPAS, PA-C; Richard D. Ball, DHSc, MPH, PAC; Jordan Beckley, MPAS, PA-C; Justina Bennett, MPAS, PA-C; James F. Cawley, MPH, PA-C Emeritus, DHL(hon); Jane S. Davis, DNP; Shea A. Dempsey, DMSc, MBA, PA-C, CAQ-EM; Jerica N. Derr, DMSc, PA-C; Christine Fuller, MHS, PA-C; Jeanine Gargiulo, MPAS, PA-C; Trisha Harris, DHA, MS, PA-C; Mary Holthaus, MSPAS, PA-C; Tia Kadiu; Gerald Kayingo, PhD, MBA, PA-C, DFAAPA; Lucy W. Kibe, DrPH, MS, MHS, PA-C; Kenneth E. Korber, PA, MHPE, DFAAPA; Brent Luu, PharmD, BCACP; Jennie McKown, MSHS, PA-C; Multak Multak, PhD, MPAS, PA-C, DFAAPA; Melissa Murfin, PharmD, BCACP, PA-C, DFAAPA; Donna Murray, DMSc, MS, PAC; Eric C. Nemec, PharmD, MEd; Laura Okolie, DMSc, MBA, MHS, PA-C; Susan M. Salahshor, PhD, PA-C, DFAAPA; Katrina M. Schrode, PhD; Sarah Schuur, PA-C, MPAS; Brittany Stokes- Francis, PA-C, MS; Victoria Trott, MMS, PA-C, AQH; Sampath Wijesinghe, DHSc, MS, MPAS, PA-C, AAHIVS; ToriAnne M. Yetter, PA-C, PMH-C, CLSP; Kim Zuber, PA-C

The Clinics staff listed below have identified no financial relationships or relationships to products or devices they have with ineligible companies related to the content of this CME activity:
Taylor Hayes; Kothainayaki Kulanthaivelu; Michelle Littlejohn; Patrick J. Manley; Anirban Mukherjee

UNAPPROVED/OFF-LABEL USE DISCLOSURE
The EOCME requires CME faculty to disclose to the participants:
1. When products or procedures being discussed are off-label, unlabelled, experimental, and/or investigational (not US Food and Drug Administration [FDA] approved); and

2. Any limitations on the information presented, such as data that are preliminary or that represent ongoing research, interim analyses, and/or unsupported opinions. Faculty may discuss information about pharmaceutical agents that is outside of FDA-approved labelling. This information is intended solely for CME and is not intended to promote off-label use of these medications. If you have any questions, contact the medical affairs department of the manufacturer for the most recent prescribing information.

TO ENROLL

The CME program is available to all *Physician Assistant Clinics* subscribers at no additional fee. To subscribe to the *Physician Assistant Clinics*, call customer service at 1-800-654-2452 or sign up online at www.physicianassistant.theclinics.com.

METHOD OF PARTICIPATION

In order to claim credit, participants must complete the following:
1. Complete enrolment as indicated above
2. Read the activity
3. Complete the CME Test and Evaluation. Participants must achieve a score of 70% on the test. All CME Tests and Evaluations must be completed online

CME INQUIRIES/SPECIAL NEEDS

For all CME inquiries or special needs, please contact elsevierCME@elsevier.com.

Contributors

CONSULTING EDITORS

KIM ZUBER, PA-C
Executive Director, American Academy of Nephrology PAs, Melbourne, Florida, USA

JANE S. DAVIS, DNP
Nurse Practitioner, Division of Nephrology, University of Alabama at Birmingham, Birmingham, Alabama, USA

EDITORS

LUCY W. KIBE, DrPH, MS, MHS, PA-C
Program Director and Associate Professor, PA Program, Charles R. Drew University of Medicine and Science, Los Angeles, California, USA

GERALD KAYINGO, PhD, MBA, PA-C, DFAAPA
Assistant Dean, Executive Director, and Professor, Physician Assistant Leadership and Learning Academy, School of Graduate Studies, University of Maryland, Baltimore, Baltimore, Maryland, USA

AUTHORS

EDWARD ADINKRAH, MD, MPH, PMP
Post-Doctoral Research Fellow, Department of Family Medicine, Charles R. Drew University of Medicine and Science, Los Angeles, California, USA

FELIX ALVELO, MPAS, PA-C
Adjunct Faculty, Department of Family Medicine, Mid Valley Clinic & Hospital, Omak, Washington, USA

RICHARD D. BALL, DHSc, MPH, PA-C
Assistant Dean/Program Director, Associate Professor, MPAS Program, Department of Medical Education, Herbert Wertheim College of Medicine, Miami, Florida, USA

JORDAN BECKLEY, MPAS, PA-C
Adjunct Faculty, CVS Minute Clinic, Washington, DC, USA; Ithaca College, Ithaca, NY, USA

JUSTINA BENNETT, MPAS, PA-C
Adjunct Faculty, Department of PA Medicine, Frostburg State University, Hagerstown, Maryland, USA

JAMES F. CAWLEY, MPH, PA-C Emeritus, DHL(Hon)
Professor and Scholar-in-Residence, Physician Assistant Leadership and Learning Academy, University of Maryland Baltimore, Baltimore, Maryland, USA; Professor Emeritus and past Chair, Department of Prevention and Community Health, Milken Institute School of Public Health, The George Washington University, Washington, DC, USA

SHEA A. DEMPSEY, DMSc, MBA, PA-C, CAQ-EM
Assistant Professor/Founding Director, Doctor of Medical Science, Shenandoah
University, Winchester, Virginia, USA

JERICA N. DERR, DMSc, PA-C
Associate Director of Research and Capstone Activities, Doctor of Medical Science
Program, Department of Physician Assistant Studies, A.T. Still University, Arizona School
of Health Sciences, Mesa, Arizona, USA; Director of Experiential Learning and Assistant
Professor, Division of Physician Assistant Education, Oregon Health & Science University
School of Medicine, Portland, Oregon, USA

KAREN FINKLEA, DMSc, PA-C
Physician Associate, Department of Obstetrics and Gynecology, Anthony L. Jordan
Health Center, Rochester, New York, USA

CHRISTINE FULLER, MHS, PA-C
PALLA Fellow, Physician Assistant Leadership and Learning Academy Graduate School,
University of Maryland, Baltimore, Baltimore, Maryland, USA

JEANINE GARGIULO, MPAS, PA-C
Assistant Professor, Physician Assistant Program, Graduate School, University of
Maryland, Baltimore, Baltimore, Maryland, USA

TRISHA HARRIS, DHA, MS, PA-C
Course Instructor, University of Maryland Eastern Shore, Princess Anne, Maryland, USA;
FCCS Course Director and Instructor, University of the Virgin Islands Medical Simulation
Center, Saint Croix, U.S. Virgin Islands

MARY HOLTHAUS, MSPAS, PA-C
Physician Assistant, Department of Neurology, Virginia Commonwealth University
Medical Center, Richmond, Virginia, USA

TEUTA KADIU, RN, PhD
Betty Irene Moore School of Nursing, UC Davis, Sacramento, California, USA

KENNETH E. KORBER, PA, MHPE, DFAAPA
Assistant Professor and Founding Faculty, Physician Assistant Training Program, Touro
University and Health System, Illinois, Skokie, Illinois, USA

BRENT LUU, PharmD, BCACP
Associate Clinical Professor, Betty Irene Moore School of Nursing, UC Davis,
Sacramento, California, USA

JENNIE McKOWN, MSHS, PA-C
Physician Assistant, Department of Surgery, The Johns Hopkins Hospital, Baltimore,
Maryland, USA

NINA MULTAK, PhD, MPAS, PA-C, DFAAPA
Professor, Associate Dean, Director School of PA Studies, University of Florida College of
Medicine, Gainesville, Florida, USA

MELISSA MURFIN, PharmD, BCACP, PA-C, DFAAPA
Program Director and Associate Professor, Physician Assistant Program, School
of Health Sciences and Human Performance, Ithaca College, Ithaca, New York,
USA

DONNA F. MURRAY, DMSc, MS, PA-C
Clinical Adjunct Professor, Morehouse School of Medicine PA Studies Program, Atlanta, Georgia, USA

ERIC C. NEMEC, PharmD, MEd
Asscoiate Professor, PA Studies, Heart University, Fairfield, Connecticut, USA

LAURA OKOLIE, DMSc, MBA, MHS, PA-C
Medical Instructor, Department of Family Medicine and Community Health, Duke University School of Medicine, Durham, North Carolina, USA

SUSAN M. SALAHSHOR, PhD, PA-C, DFAAPA
Associate Professor, Department of Arts and Sciences, Ottawa University, Overland Park, Kansas, USA

KATRINA M. SCHRODE, PhD
Assistant Professor, Department of Psychiatry, Charles R. Drew University of Medicine and Science, Los Angeles, California, USA

SARAH SCHUUR, PA-C, MPAS
Research Fellow, Physician Assistant Leadership and Learning Academy, Graduate School, University of Maryland, Baltimore, Baltimore, Maryland, USA

BRITTANY STOKES-FRANCIS, PA-C, MS
Clinical Assistant Professor, Department of Physician Assistant, Howard University, Washington, DC, USA

VICTORIA TROTT, MMS, PA-C, AQH
Director of Advocacy and Leadership Development, Physician Assistant Leadership and Learning Academy, Physician Assistant, Department of Neurosurgery, University of Maryland, Baltimore, Maryland, USA

SAMPATH WIJESINGHE, DHSc, MS, MPAS, PA-C, AAHIVS
Clinical Associate Professor, School of Medicine, Stanford University, Stanford, California, USA

TORIANNE M. YETTER, DMS, PA-C, PMH-C, CLSP
Physician Assistant, Department of Family Medicine, ChristianaCare, Newark DE, USA

Contents

The digital transformation of health care has been evolving, with the pivotal point in history for the technological revolution in health care occurring in 2020 when the coronavirus 2019 pandemic forced the world to develop new ways to remain connected to patients and to continue patient care despite mandated isolation and quarantine practices. Today, the use of media and other technological platforms to learn has grown exponentially. This holds true for patient education as well. When discussing the digital transformation of patient education, one must include the challenges and barriers that may be faced by the clinician and the patient. The technological revolution in health care and specifically, patient education is occurring, and the outlook and benefits are promising.

As self-directed learners, physician assistants are familiar with the notion that continuing professional development keeps us plugged into the advances of medicine and surgery and is part of our patient advocacy's "secret sauce." However, when it comes to our patient's perspective, they may not know what they don't know—despite patient education being part of our health advocacy goals. Therein lays a clinical challenge. We explore the role of health literacy and special patient education situations where effective communication is tantamount to better health outcomes.

"Empowering Patients through Health Information" is a comprehensive guide designed to enhance patient access and understanding of health information, fostering informed decision-making in the health care context. It addresses the challenges of misinformation and the importance of health information privacy and security. Strategies for health care providers to facilitate patient health literacy are emphasized, including critical evaluation of health information, and safeguarding digital health data. The significance of cultural and ethical considerations in patient education and empowerment in the digital health era is also discussed.

Healthcare literacy is a driving force that could improve health outcomes. In order for patients to obtain, process, and understand the basic health information, education must be provided by clinicians from various disciplines. A team-based approach (TBA) to patient education must be developed and considered to enhance the diversity of the provided educational information. TBA to patient education requires the collaboration of different professionals within health care system to improve patient outcomes such as reduction of preventable adverse drug reactions, increased therapeutic optimization, or decreased morbidity and mortality.

This article explores the intricate interplay between health equity and social justice recognizing the profound impact of social determinants and health care disparities on the health and well-being of the population of the United States. Understanding the complexity of the intersection of health equity and social justice provides the clarity needed to recognize the urgent need for collaborative efforts among health care professionals, policymakers, and communities to dismantle structural barriers and advance a vision of health equity grounded in social justice principles.

This article explores the role of educating patients in managing chronic diseases, and stresses its value in aiding lifestyle modifications, adhering to medication regimens, and self-management. By exploring proven methods, technological tools for health, and helpful tips for health professionals, this article demonstrates the varied influence patient education has on chronic disease management. Key points also addressed highlight the success of interventions in enhancing patient understanding, engagement, and adherence to treatment regimens while tackling such challenges as health literacy levels, limited access to resources, and cultural sensitivity.

The sequela of hospitalization frequently entails many changes for patients. A primary goal of health care is to educate patients so they are empowered to be shared decision-makers related to their care. Patient education is a complex function of providing information coupled with the patient's ability to understand, frequently called health literacy. This article describes evidence-based strategies to enhance patient education in the hospital setting. It is structured similarly to an inpatient encounter, encompasses best practices, and culminates in a case study.

It is essential that health care professionals develop skills and competencies on how to provide effective patient education to enhance health outcomes, improve patient experience, and reduce costs while enhancing quality and safety. This article presents the current evidence-based practices on patient education for preventative health care. The article summarizes historical trends, theoretic frameworks, barriers and provides tools for the clinician to use in practice.

Patient education during clinical interactions helps to improve health behaviors and clinical outcomes. The focus of the article involves the following special populations: intellectually disabled, developmentally disabled, and geriatric/older adults. Patient education approaches in these subpopulations vary in terms of health concerns, best practices, and strategies. However, there are commonalities within these subpopulations regarding health literacy, challenges, and future directions. The La Trobe Support for Decision-making Practice Framework for the intellectually and developmentally disabled populations and the comprehensive geriatric assessment for the geriatric population are discussed as recommendations for best practice to identify the needs of these corresponding patient populations.

Perinatal mental health has primarily taken the backseat to the physiologic bodily conditions of the pregnant person, especially in marginalized populations. While obstetric and reproductive psychiatry may not be readily available in many settings, the primary care provider is frequently front line. Physicians and advanced practice clinicians (APCs) have the unique opportunity to familiarize themselves and become comfortable with identifying a perinatal patient at risk for perinatal mental health disorders. With appropriate education of the APC and, in turn, the patient, clinicians may also play a vital role in the management of perinatal mood and anxiety disorders, thus lowering postpartum comorbidity.

Every clinician should assess patient education and content delivery to determine effectiveness. This article discusses the theoretic foundations of patient education, its establishment, and its transformation over the years. It examines modern patient education challenges, such as limited appointment times and health literacy with diverse populations. The article concludes with current evidence-based assessment tools and future directions to improve patient education.

Precision medicine, or personalized medicine, has opened the door to a better understanding of individualizing patient care. Genetic and genomic testing is an important tool that allows for diagnosis of genetic conditions and guiding treatment recommendations when genetic variants are present. Patient education includes helping patients understand when a genetic test is needed, the meaning of the results, and how the results may help determine appropriate treatment. Ethical considerations around education of patients undergoing genetic testing include informed consent for the patient, notification of family in the case of inherited conditions, and storage and use of the patients' genetic materials.

The rising cost of health care in the United States has impacted access and exacerbated health care disparities particularly in low-income and medium-income communities. Effective health education has the potential to prevent disease, promote wellness, cut costs, and promote health equity. This study explores the intricate relationship between health education and health care economics. It delves into the financial aspects of patient education, including billing, coding, group education, and the substantial savings that can be realized through the prevention of diseases and hospitalizations.

Preparing physician assistant/associate (PA) students to provide patient education is an underdeveloped area of curricula. Patient education is made up of both science and the art of conveying medical knowledge. Much like any human interaction, the process of providing patient education is complex and encompasses many skills in the affective learning domain including the development of emotional intelligence, which is an essential competency for effective patient education. When there is human interaction, there is an emotional aspect. Developing, teaching, and assessing these skills have proven to be a challenge in PA education and warrant further attention and development of strategies.

As more patients become actively involved in their care, there has been an evolution toward thorough patient education. Patients and their advocates have pushed against a one-size-fits-all approach and instead desire a customized experience. An important current trend in health care that professionals must consider is medical decisions are becoming more standardized and codified. With this realization, it is important to be intentional with patient education and not base it or medical decision-making exclusively on formal guidelines. Decisions and directives need to be individualized, especially when they involve choices between possible outcomes that may be viewed differently by different patients.

Shea A. Dempsey and Karen Finklea

As health care evolves, several innovative opportunities to improve patient education in the twenty-first century have been created. The core competencies of physician assistant/associate (PA) education include patient education and advanced educational credentials have the potential to enhance these competencies and better prepare PAs for the ever-evolving health care climate. This article explores how the PA profession can leverege Advanced credentionals to improve patient education and optimize patient care.

Advances in Patient Education: An Integrated Approach
PHYSICIAN ASSISTANT CLINICS

FORTHCOMING ISSUES

January 2025
Neurology
Amy Dix, *Editor*

April 2025
Cardiology
Sondra DePalma, *Editor*

July 2025
Urology
Molly Elizabeth Band and Victor
Quintanilla, *Editors*

RECENT ISSUES

July 2024
Gender Minority Medicine
Diane Bruessow, *Editor*

April 2024
Medicine Outside Four Walls
Kim Zuber and Jane S. Davis, *Editors*

January 2024
General Orthopedics
Kara-Ann Valentine, *Editor*

SERIES OF RELATED INTEREST

Primary Care: Clinics in Office Practice
https://www.primarycare.theclinics.com/
Medical Clinics
https://www.medical.theclinics.com/

THE CLINICS ARE AVAILABLE ONLINE!
Access your subscription at:
www.theclinics.com

Foreword

The Destination: Optimum Patient Care; The Travelers: Patients and Providers; The Bridge: Education

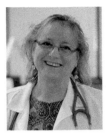 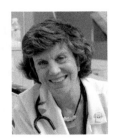

Kim Zuber, PA-C   Jane S. Davis, DNP
Consulting Editors

Lucy W. Kibe and Gerald Kayingo, both leaders in Physician Assistant/Associate (PA) professional education, bring together experts from across the field on the value and techniques of patient education.

When patients understand the why, they often are more willing and able to follow the providers' suggestions. This involves going to where a patient is (think health literacy or numeracy) and the patient's needs. These can be social or economic needs but also learning style. The editors, through selection of their incredible authors, introduce us to utilizing technology to our advantage and adjusting our teaching strategies for different populations and settings. No matter how well we educate PAs for the twenty-first century, if they cannot explain the what, the how, or the why to a patient, all the training in the world has been wasted.

Education does not happen in a vacuum. One can design the best outreach, but if the community does not understand the education outreach, it is useless. True understanding occurs when the lessons fit the culture, and we all follow directions we understand. The authors guide us in techniques to evaluate and improve our effectiveness.

As each patient has opportunities to interact with multiple health care providers, the authors include a team approach for patient benefit. Everyone on the team is important, and everyone has a part to deliver and to reinforce the others' directions.

In a rapidly changing world where the latest technique is soon displaced by something newer and better, it is essential to be mindful of the ethics of education when utilizing some tools and technologies.

The PA, through training and education, is uniquely positioned to be at the forefront of patient care and education. This too is explored in the Education issue of *Physician Assistant Clinics*.

Physician Assist Clin 9 (2024) xv–xvi
https://doi.org/10.1016/j.cpha.2024.07.002
2405-7991/24/© 2024 Published by Elsevier Inc.
physicianassistant.theclinics.com

We think all PAs will find this issue beneficial. We hope it is one that will increase effectiveness of patient education, patient satisfaction, and positive health outcomes. We suspect it will.

DISCLOSURES

The authors have no conflicts of interest to disclose.

Kim Zuber, PA-C
American Academy of Nephrology PAs
Melbourne, FL, USA

Jane S. Davis, DNP
Division of Nephrology
University of Alabama at Birmingham
Birmingham, AL, USA

E-mail addresses:
zuberkim@yahoo.com (K. Zuber)
jsdavis@uabmc.edu (J.S. Davis)

Preface

Physician Assistants at the Forefront of Patient Education

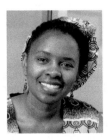 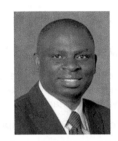

Lucy W. Kibe, DrPH, MS, MHS, PA-C   Gerald Kayingo, PhD, MBA, PA-C, DFAAPA

Editors

In the ever-evolving landscape of health care, patient education stands as a cornerstone for fostering informed and empowered individuals. As we continue to practice in a new era in medicine, where collaborative and patient-centered care is key, the need for advancing patient education has never been more critical. This series, "Advances in Patient Education: An Integrated Approach," delves into the critical facets of patient education, presenting a comprehensive exploration of innovative strategies and advancements that are shaping the future of health care communication.

SIGNIFICANCE OF THE ISSUE

Patient education has transcended its traditional role, emerging as a pivotal force in shaping health care experiences. The contemporary health care landscape demands a paradigm shift toward an integrated approach that considers the multifaceted dimensions of patient education.

WHAT READERS WILL FIND IN THIS SERIES

This series brings together a diverse collection of insights from experts and practitioners at the forefront of patient care and education. Structured to cover a spectrum of topics, this issue explores the role of technology, health care team dynamics, and

Physician Assist Clin 9 (2024) xvii–xix

https://doi.org/10.1016/j.cpha.2024.06.001

2405-7991/24/© 2024 Published by Elsevier Inc.

physicianassistant.theclinics.com

the training of Physician Assistant (PA) students in fostering a patient-centered approach.

Each article delves into innovative methods, case studies, and emerging trends, starting with the current challenges in patient education and offering practical solutions. Topics include the use of digital health tools, the impact of cultural competence on patient communication, and the transformative potential of advanced education for health care providers. The inclusion of diverse perspectives serves to enrich the discourse and inspire health care practitioners to embrace innovative strategies in their own patient education endeavors.

TAKEAWAYS AND IMPLICATIONS

As readers engage with the content presented in this series, they will gain a nuanced understanding of the transformative potential of an integrated approach to patient education. The takeaways are manifold:

1. Real-world applications: Practical applications and success stories highlight the real-world impact of advanced education programs, demonstrating their relevance in diverse health care settings.
2. Adaptability in practice: The series underscores the adaptability of PAs, showcasing how they can evolve to meet the evolving needs of patients, the health care system, and evolving technologies.
3. Future directions: The discussions extend beyond the present, offering a glimpse into the future of patient education. Readers will be equipped to anticipate and embrace forthcoming changes in health care delivery.

CLOSING THOUGHTS

"Advances in Patient Education: An Integrated Approach" is not merely a compilation of theories; it is a testament to the ongoing evolution of health care education. Through its pages, readers will embark on a journey beyond conventional boundaries, embracing a future where patient education is not just informative but transformative. It is our sincere hope that this series will serve as a catalyst for positive change, fostering a culture where informed and engaged patients are at the heart of a healthier tomorrow.

ACKNOWLEDGMENT OF REVIEWERS

The editors would like to acknowledge the following individuals who participated in reviewing the manuscripts. Candra Carr, MS, PA-C; Cara Felter, PT, PhD, DPT, MPH; Colleen Ohm, MMS, PA-C; Cynthia Griffith, MPAS, PA-C; Hyun-Jin Jun, PhD, MSW; Laurarose Dunn-O'Farrell, PA-C, LCPC; Margarita Loeza, MD, MPH; Natalie Houser,

DMSc, PA-C; Nicole Reichhart, MPAS, PA-C; Orette Clarke, MD, MBS; Shani Fleming, PhD, MSHS, MPH, PA-C.

DISCLOSURES

The Guest Editors have nothing to disclose.

Lucy W. Kibe, DrPH, MS, MHS
PA-CPA Program
Charles R. Drew University of Science and Health
College of Science and Health
1731 East 120th Street
Los Angeles, CA 90059, USA

Gerald Kayingo, PhD, MBA, PA-C, DFAAPA
Physician Assistant Leadership and Learning Academy
School of Graduate Studies
University of Maryland, Baltimore
520 West Fayette Street, Suite #130
Baltimore, MD 21201, USA

E-mail addresses:
lucykibe@cdrewu.edu (L.W. Kibe)
gkayingo@umaryland.edu (G. Kayingo)

The Role of Technology in Patient Education

Christine Fuller, MHS, PA-C[a,*], Nina Multak, PhD, MPAS, PA-C, DFAAPA[b]

KEYWORDS

- Patient education • Digital transformation • Telemedicine • Digital health
- Digital literacy • Healthcare technology

KEY POINTS

- Despite the technological advancement of health care, the digital transformation of patient health education is in the beginning stages of evolution.
- The types of technology used for patient education encompass a wide range of modalities that are currently in practice and are actively being developed.
- Challenges and barriers to the evolution of patient education are to be considered and discussed along with solutions to ensure optimal outcomes.
- The ethical and legal aspects associated with the advancement in the transformation of patient education require addressing to provide and protect patients as well as the health care system globally.
- The clinician's role in providing appropriate patient education during the digital transformation of health care is critical to ensure that the best outcomes can be achieved for all of the moving parts in the process of delivery and receipt of care.

INTRODUCTION

Overview

Patient education is a vital part of health care services as patients and proxy medical decision makers have become more involved in a symbiotic approach to the diagnosis and treatment of clinical conditions and injuries. The methods and modalities utilized to deliver instructions and care plans to patients have changed through the years with the most recent evolution being the digital transformation of patient education. According to Angelos I. Stoumpos, and colleagues, article titled "Digital Transformation in Healthcare: Technology Acceptance and Its Applications,"[1] digital transformation is the ongoing process of change made using digital technology to benefit society. In health care, this includes but is not limited to changes using digital technology and

[a] PALLA, University of Maryland Baltimore, 520 West Fayette Street, First Floor, Baltimore, MD 21201, USA; [b] University of Florida College of Medicine, PO Box 100176, Gainesville, FL 32610, USA
* Corresponding author. 520 West Fayette Street, First Floor, Baltimore, MD 21201.
E-mail address: christine.wentt@umm.edu

Physician Assist Clin 9 (2024) 467–478
https://doi.org/10.1016/j.cpha.2024.05.001
2405-7991/24/© 2024 Elsevier Inc. All rights are reserved, including those for text and data mining, AI training, and similar technologies.

the internet throughout the entire health care process with hopes of improving patient outcomes. The interaction between patient and provider plays a vital role in patient health outcome and patient education has been an integral part of this interaction. Through the digital transformation of health care, patient education has had to evolve as well. Much has been discussed about the impact and evolution of the health care industry with regards to its digital transformation; however, impact on patient education has not been a topic in the forefront and much research into the application, implication, and ramification of digital transformation is needed. This text will visit the digital transformation of patient education including the history, current landscape, theoretic foundations, best practices, and ethical, cultural, diversity, and existing challenges that may be faced, as well as future direction and opportunities.

Objectives

By the end of this article, the reader will be able to.

- Discuss digital transformation with regards to patient education.
- Describe strategies that are utilized in the delivery and implementation of patient education with regards to advancing uses of technology.
- Summarize the advantages and disadvantages of the digital transformation of patient education.
- Identify ethical and legal challenges and barriers to patient care because of digital transformation in health care.
- Recognize some issues with diversity and inclusion of patients with regards to patient education as health care delivery evolves through digital transformation.

Key Concepts

Digital transformation, patient education, telemedicine, mobile medicine, simulation, electronic learning, digital literacy.

BACKGROUND AND CONTEXT
History

Patient education encourages patients to become active participants in their own health by developing an in-depth understanding of their care plans, increased adherence, and improved efficiency through facilitating patient-clinician discussions. Patients used to receive information and education by way of teaching directly from nurses after the clinician had diagnosed and developed a treatment plan for them. Educating patients has been part of patient care from the beginning of structured health care. According to writing from Bella J. May, EdD, PT, FAPTA titled, "Patient Education: Past and Present,"[2] around 1315, French surgeons were required to "inform patients of risks" of surgery before incision was made. This was the first Civil Chamber of the Court of Cassation.[2] Around the end of World War II, as people in the United States began living longer, clinicians began to diagnose and treat more chronic illnesses and conditions. As a result, there was a shift in the focus to educate patients on the management of these chronic illnesses and conditions.

In the past, patient education was geared toward instruction on self-care and consent for procedures as it was thought that medical language, ideas, and practice were too technical to give to patients and expect comprehension. Patients were educated on diet, activity, how to take medications, and wound care.[1–3] The actual procedure and reason behind the medical treatment was not fully disclosed at those times. Patients just did as they were expected to do with what they were told as practitioners were viewed as authority figures.

Patient education was also in the form of prescriptions and verbal instructions post World War II. The change came around 1950 to 1960.[2] With research demonstrating that people wanted to learn about the illnesses and conditions that they suffered, patient education changed forever. Today, we stress patient education as patients have taken a role in their own outcomes and responsibility for their own health. The way education is delivered has significantly changed, evolving from verbal instruction, prescriptions, and consent to more technologically sound forms of education which includes paper format to online digital formats. The present and future of patient education has and will change the face of health care in this country.

The pivot point in patient education from verbal instruction, prescription, and consent to paper gradually occurred and patients were expected to read pamphlets as well as remember what was spoken to them. Although effective in capturing many patients by allowing them to review written material, the world was changing technologically, and all aspects of health care are required to adapt to this change. In the year 2020, a critical event occurred that changed the health care models we, as a people, had grown accustomed to in the United States.[4] The country, along with the entire world, experienced a phenomenon that caused unprecedented change in the life of every individual and the way we practiced in health care and in educating patients. The coronavirus disease 2019 (COVID-19) pandemic caused by severe acute respiratory syndrome coronavirus 2, resulted in a quarantine and reverse quarantine type of policy in this country which forced health care practices to drastically change whether we were ready or not. Technology was required to be used as this is included in patient education. There was a rush to figure out how to remain in contact with patients and their families while practicing evidence-based medicine while maintaining standards of care.[5]

Technology has increased the speed in information availability and current utilization of health-related information. Patient education has come a long way from the time when patients solely relied on health care providers when seeking information about their medical condition and instructions on effective management—both pharmacologic and nonpharmacologic. Currently, patients, as well as their caregivers, are increasingly relying on Google searches (and Siri/Alexa) to resolve their health care-related inquiries. Health care practitioners are no longer the only source of information that patients can rely on. Making use of technology to bridge the gap between the patients and health care providers and providing them with relevant and reliable information through patient education is of paramount importance to ensure quality health care delivery and improved patient outcomes.[4–8]

E-learning and online resources: multimedia resources

An advantage of well-designed multimedia for patient education is flexibility. Multimedia can assist clinicians in overcoming linguistic, cultural, and physical barriers, addressing different learning levels, presenting materials in different formats and from different perspectives; in providing feedback and decision-making resources; and in tailoring and customizing information to the needs of individual patients and providers. It is only within the educational, cognitive, cultural, clinical, social, ethical, financial, and personal landscape that user preference emerges and the value of multimedia can truly be evaluated.[9–11]

Examples

- MedlinePlus: Videos & Tools
    MedlinePlus contains operating room (OR)-Live surgery videos, interactive patient education tutorials and images from government and contracted

sources.[8,12] To search for an image, type in image topic and "image" (ex. "heart image" (no quotes) to find images of hearts). To search for a video, type in video topic and "video" (ex. bariatric surgery video). Governmentally produced information is not copyrighted; however, selected images videos (as well as some other content in MedlinePlus) do have copyright restrictions. For copyright and use information for each content publisher, visit the MedlinePlus copyright information page. To get directly to the video/tutorial content, scroll down on the site map and select between Interactive Health Tutorials, Surgery Videos, or Anatomy videos.

- WebMD: Slideshows, Quizzes and Assessments A to Z
  Browse slides by health topic from A to Z.

Technology Can Enhance Patient Education in Several Ways, Including

- Personalization: Providing personalized and interactive content.
- Access: Improving access and convenience.
- Communication: Facilitating communication and feedback.
- Convenience: Offering many of the same amenities that consumers use at home.

Examples of Patient Education Technology Include

- E-learning and online resources
- Patient portals for education via telemedicine
- Visualization through 3-dimensional printing technology
- Simulation-based patient education apps

Mobile Applications for Patient Education

Apps for patient education

1. Applications or apps are software programs designed to accomplish a particular purpose, with an increasing number of apps focused on health care.[13] The world of health care app development has fostered a rich ecosystem of applications, each tailored to address specific needs within the health care sector. These ingenious apps are engineered to elevate patient outcomes, streamline health care delivery, and empower individuals to actively manage their well-being.

2. Apps focused on health care can be used for tasks such as sending reminders to take medications, providing education, or enabling a person to record blood pressure measurements. Health apps are commonly used on mobile devices such as smartphones (eg, an iPhone or Android), tablets (eg, iPad), and smartwatches (eg, Apple Watch or FitBit). Smartwatches are devices that run apps and are worn on the wrist. These devices are called wearables.

3. Health care apps are personalized for specific type of end-user. Patient-facing apps are directed at the patient for the purpose of self-care, which can include education or information about general wellness or specific disease states. Some apps function to direct patient self-care that involves monitoring health status (ie, monitoring blood sugar levels) or treatment that directs the patient to take specific actions for addressing their own health (ie, medication adherence). Clinician-facing apps provide medical education or information from a treatment perspective. These apps may assist with diagnosis of a disease or help clinicians advise appropriate preventive care (ie, calculating stroke risk factor scores). Some health care apps are a hybrid between patient-facing and clinician-facing and function to communicate between patient and clinician (ie, patient-measured vital signs are recorded and communicated to the clinician through the app).[8] The recent increase in

the demand for digital health care will likely precipitate continued research with user feedback providing innovation in health care app design.
4. An area of health care app design that needs to be addressed is equity. App end users, particularly those in marginalized groups, who have low health literacy or low levels of experience with technology, might have difficulty using these apps. This situation is further compounded by issues with limited access to WiFi or a device such as a smartphone or tablet. A lack of reliable access to technology components creates potential for harm among patients who then may not be able to access care provided through these apps and could further widen care disparities. App evaluation frameworks that include equity considerations should be prioritized in the app design process.[8]

What Is the Difference Between a Health App and a Medical App?

The terms "health app" and "medical app" are often used interchangeably, but there are distinct differences between them.

Health Apps: Health apps are designed to promote general wellness, healthy habits, and self-care. They focus on empowering individuals to make informed decisions about their well-being. Health apps provide features and functionalities that help users track and manage various aspects of their health, such as physical activity, nutrition, sleep patterns, stress levels, and mindfulness.

These apps typically offer tools for activity tracking, exercise routines, calorie counting, meditation exercises, and personalized health tips. Health apps aim to enhance overall wellness, encourage healthy lifestyles, and empower individuals to take proactive steps toward better health. They may also offer educational resources, articles, and community support related to general health and wellness.

Medical Apps: Medical apps are specifically designed to provide health care-related services, diagnosis, treatment, and support. These apps are developed with the involvement of health care professionals and are subject to more stringent regulations and certifications. Medical apps focus on delivering clinical information, aiding in diagnosis, managing medical conditions, and facilitating health care provider-patient interactions, including patient education.

Medical apps often require approval from regulatory bodies, such as the Food and Drug Administration in the United States, to ensure their safety and effectiveness. They may offer functionalities like secure messaging with health care providers, access to electronic health records, medication reminders, remote monitoring of health conditions, and specialized tools for health care professionals.[14–16]

Examples of Medical Apps

- *Telemedicine Apps:* Telemedicine apps have revolutionized the way health care is delivered by providing remote access to medical professionals.[14–18] These apps enable patients to connect with health care providers through video consultations, voice calls, or secure messaging. Telemedicine apps have gained immense popularity, especially in recent times, as they offer convenience, reduce the need for in-person visits, and expand access to health care services, particularly for individuals in rural or remote areas. This enhances opportunities for patient education.
- *Appointment Scheduling and Patient Portal Apps:* These apps simplify the process of booking appointments, allowing patients to schedule, reschedule, or cancel appointments at their convenience. Patient portal apps also provide access to medical records, lab results, prescription history, and other essential health information. By empowering patients with convenient self-service options,

these apps streamline administrative tasks, enhance patient engagement, and improve overall patient experience.

- *Medication Management Apps:* Medication management apps help individuals track their medication schedules, set reminders for taking medications, and provide information about drug interactions and potential side effects. These apps can also facilitate prescription refills and send notifications to health care providers or caregivers to ensure medication adherence. By promoting medication safety and adherence, medication management apps play a crucial role in preventing medication errors and improving treatment outcomes.
- *Fitness and Wellness Apps*: Fitness and wellness apps promote healthy lifestyles by offering features such as activity tracking, exercise routines, nutrition tracking, sleep monitoring, and mindfulness exercises. These apps enable users to set health goals, track their progress, and receive personalized recommendations for improving their overall well-being. Fitness and wellness apps empower individuals to take charge of their health, make informed decisions, and adopt healthier habits.
- *Chronic Disease Management Apps:* Chronic disease management apps cater to individuals living with chronic conditions such as diabetes, hypertension, asthma, or arthritis. These apps allow users to monitor symptoms, track vital signs, record medications, and log lifestyle factors that impact their condition. They can provide insights, trends, and reminders to help users manage their condition effectively. Chronic disease management apps empower patients to actively participate in their care, improve self-management, and achieve better health outcomes.
- *Mental Health and Mindfulness Apps:* Mental health and mindfulness apps offer tools and resources to support mental well-being. These apps provide meditation exercises, stress management techniques, mood tracking, and therapy resources. They promote relaxation, reduce anxiety, and enhance emotional well-being. Mental health apps contribute to breaking down the stigma surrounding mental health and provide accessible support for those in need.

Current Landscape

As patient education continues to evolve and has undergone a digital transformation, we must look at current modalities and methods which can be used to educate patients. Verbal instruction and printed paper information continues to be utilized, however, a pivotal moment in patient education was the rise of the internet.[19,20] The internet has created a gateway to sharing information and knowledge from anywhere in the world. This includes patient education being shared. Most of the people within the United States have access to the internet via the cell phone and for that reason the access to patient education has been allowed to expand the borders of the clinic. Patients are being reached through online health information, social media platforms such as Facebook, X (formerly Twitter), and LinkedIn. In the past 20 years, according to a review by Sravya Chirumamilla and Martha Gulati titled "Patient Education and Engagement through Social Media"[3] from 2019, use of social media as a source of gathering information has significantly increased. With the digital era of information sharing, factors that govern the type of platform utilized for patient education will vary widely. The factors include but are not limited to race, sex, socioeconomic status, and generation or age of the user. For example, the digital media platforms Snapchat, TikTok, and Instagram are used by a younger generation, those under 24 year old, whereas LinkedIn are utilized more by those with college degrees and with higher incomes.[3] When selecting which platform to use for patient education, the demographics of the patient must be considered. This can offer a challenge in the standardization of patient education for health care organizations and providers alike.

Unlike social media platforms for patient education, the use of simulation to educate patients with acute or chronic illnesses is new. The utilization of simulation-based education, however, is not a new concept and has been in practice in teaching health care professionals for quite some time. According to an article by Abdulmohsen H. Al-Elq from the Department of Internal Medicine at the College of Medicine, University of Dammam in Saudi Arabia titled "Simulation-based Medical Teaching and Learning,"[21] simulation-based medical teaching can be defined as the artificial representation of real-world clinical scenarios used in medical teaching through experiential learning. The development and use of simulation in education of health care professionals is expensive, however. This same modality of learning can be applied to educating patients. The use of simulation-based education for the patient learner has many challenges and according to Christelle Pennecot, PhD, et al in published study titled "Consensus Recommendations for the Use of Simulation in Therapeutic Patient Education,"[22] caution should be used when deciding to offer simulation as a tool in patient education. Not only would the cost, location, equipment, and skill development needed to use the equipment have to be accounted for, but also the ethical component such as inclusivity and biases related to patient education modality development and patient privacy must be considered. With the advancement of virtual reality in medical education, there is promising data that suggest that this modality may benefit patients when incorporated with patient education. In the journal review by Marijke van der Linde-van den Bora, et. Al, titled "The use of virtual reality in patient education related to medical somatic treatment: A scoping review,"[23] the consensus was that patients had decreased anxiety, pain, and stress and had overall improvement in preparation for treatments and in patient satisfaction rates. The utilization of virtual reality for patient education may be applied to many different populations and socioeconomic backgrounds; however, the same challenges seen with social media can apply to this use.[23]

Artificial intelligence, also called AI, is being introduced in health care. As this is an innovative technology with regards to health care, it is in the process of being discussed, developed, and used to assist in reducing workloads, improve accuracy and efficiency of work, and to assist in patient information and education. There are many forms of AI being introduced and the field is rapidly growing. The use of AI large language models is being explored as a modality to educate patients; however, this has not seemed to have been implemented as of the writing of this article.[24–27]

Challenges and considerations

The speed at which digital transformation in health care is occurring brings up major concerns not about if we are able to but rather should we proceed without having difficult conversations regarding the ethical and legal cost of such advancement in technology. Moreover, additional research will be needed to evaluate the efficacy of utilizing the different platforms and modalities with regards to the impact of the challenges faced when discussing the overall outcome of patient health because of the use of such education modalities. Some of these challenges include but are not limited to access to the different technologies, education level of the user and ability to comprehend instruction for use, comfort of the user with advanced technologies, and mental capacity of the user.

Ethics and Legal

Let us begin with the ethical and legal cost of these advanced technologies. The saying, just because we could does not mean we should, sometimes comes to mind. Yes, the technology is available, however, the ramifications of using these to generate new ways of teaching patients to care for their own illness while out of the health care setting, that is, home environment, may be far worse than if the newly developed modality had not been developed. There are issues with standardization of the information being relayed to patients on a platform which has increased the risk of being compromised by outside influences. Today, cyber security is a significant concern. Protecting patient information has been a vital part of health care practices including electronic medical records, information sharing among providers and necessary staff, and the use of electronic devices including computers and cellphones. As the information becomes more readily accessible to patients, the risk of misinformation increases. Patients and families today have access to their own personal medical records in the palm of their hands. What are the safeguards to protect the information from being altered or protect the patient from having personal information released to the public?

Human Interactions

Another challenge is the need for human interaction and touch. With the pivotal point in the digital transformation of patient education being viewed as the COVID-19 pandemic, the isolation mandated by the officials in the World Health Organization and the Center for Disease Control among other agencies resulted in widespread mental health illnesses that are still being felt today. A study conducted in Japan evaluated the mental health of adults who were in face-to-face contact versus nonface to face contact situations stemming from the pandemic (Fujiwara, and colleagues).[28] It was concluded that those who maintained face to face contact had better self-reported mental health outcomes than those who were engaged in nonface-to-face contact environments.[13] The significance of this study is to demonstrate a challenge to the digital transformation of patient education. As technology advances, the opportunity for face-to-face contact seems to decrease and therefore there is concern that the mental health of the population may decline as well. For example, an older patient with multiple comorbidities and limited mobility who resides alone may need face-to-face contact to maintain a healthy mental state and frequent visits.[29,30]

Access, Digital Literacy, and Impairments

Patient access, comprehension, and disabilities/impairments are additional factors that contribute to the challenges and barriers that clinicians will encounter when determining the modality of patient education to utilize in this advancing digital era of health care.[28,29] Although many may have access to the internet, cellular phones, and computers, there are still many without this access and knowing the population of practice may not be enough to prevent those without from having less favorable outcomes. According to the study, "Patient Experiences with Virtual Care During the COVID-19 Pandemic: Phenomenological Focus Group Study" by Curran, Hollett, and Peddle,[31] some barriers and challenges are related to the cost, access, and digital literacy which was seen in rural areas and among older populations. The cost of maintaining the availability of access to patient education in lower socioeconomic populations must be addressed. The cost of equipment, internet services, cellular phone services will be incurred by the patient who, with already costly medical needs along with basic living expenses, may become unobtainable leading to a disconnect in the traditional medical model with patient education being the bridge between good and poor overall patient outcomes. Individuals in rural communities often have scattered cell phone/internet services and the lifestyle may not rely on the use of digital technology as much as those in urban settings.[31] Also, those who do not utilize digital technology frequently may develop digital illiteracy. This lack in digital literacy would need to be corrected before the use of digital technology to educate patients can be established. Questions on the ability and availability should be asked by providers and then the platform used may be selected. Information provided to patients should be understood by the patient and available for future retrieval in order to maintain effective self-care. Considerations should include the unfamiliar language and new medical terminology that will be used. A high level of knowledge has a positive influence on patient outcomes and satisfaction.[26] However, when practicing in settings where there is a push to standardize the modality used to educate patients, this can be difficult as the resources may become restricted leaving certain populations of patients without proper and effective education opportunities, resulting in suboptimal patient outcomes.[32]

Example Case

For example, a farmer in rural America may not rely on a digital platform that the health education is presented on for day-to-day work, and therefore may not understand how to access and utilize the education that he is to receive for his insulin-dependent diabetes mellitus type II, chronic kidney disease stage III with difficult to control hypertension, peripheral vascular disease with chronic wounds. Without continued education and follow-up, the outcome for such a patient would not be optimal. To ensure that the patient who has been requesting an appointment almost weekly due to "not feeling well" and has had multiple hospitalizations gets the proper patient education and services needed for continued care and disease management at home, additional modalities may be required.

Health Care Provider and Institution Challenges and Self-Efficacy

Who would be responsible to ensure that patients improve in digital literacy, have optimal access to technology and equipment, and are able to remain connected to services while at home? Who would cover the cost? Without services in place, patients' illnesses may worsen, the overall health care cost increases, and the burden on health care resources will continue to strain the system. Although there has been progress in ensuring access, improving literacy, and subsidizing cost, there are many more who are in need. The speed at which the development and implementation of digital technology into health care, namely patient education, has surpassed the speed at which the barriers and challenges are being addressed. Care must be used to meet the patient where they are and then gradually move them forward during this digital revolution. The patient will have to be evaluated for self-efficacy to determine the patients' ability to contribute through his or her own actions to impact his or her own health status. Empowering the patient to contribute to his or her own medical decision-making process including treatment and management results in improved patient satisfaction, compliance, and perception of risks and benefits of treatments.[20] The benefit of the new modalities of patient education must not be undermined by the challenges and barriers but rather new strategies must be developed to ensure that the patient receives what is needed to ensure that optimal use, benefit, and outcome is achieved.[20]

SUMMARY

The Institute of Medicine recognizes "patient-centered care" as one of the domains of health care quality. Patient-centered care integrates the disease and illness and considers the whole patient as an individual to create a sharing of power, responsibility, and therapeutic alliance. The desire for more information on a particular subject matter is expressed verbally or in active information-seeking to assist in patients taking better care of themselves. Better understanding of patient information needs is important for providing patients with current and relevant information to assist in making informed decisions concerning their health care and allows patients to be involved in assessing health care options available to them.[33]

The digital transformation of health care is inevitable. The benefits are vast and far reaching as imaginable. Technology in health care has opened doors to allow for improvement in health care access, reliability, efficiency, and accuracy. Patient satisfaction and adherence to medical treatment has demonstrated overall improvement. However, its role in patient education is new and rapidly evolving. The duty of the clinician will be to know the audience and select the appropriate modality for their needs. The many challenges and barriers that are present within any given population cannot be discussed in this article alone. The pace of evolution outpaces the amount of research that is available on this topic in the United States. This, unfortunately, will lead to clinicians making the decision on patient education modalities without standardization and attempting to follow up closely with struggling patients to provide optimal patient outcomes. For example, there is a push for a transitional level of care that follows up with patients who are at higher risk of readmission to hospitals due to the chronicity and severity of illnesses and the compliance or number of prior admissions of patients. However, again, patient education delivery is paramount to even this service working in the patient's overall health outcome. The hopes going forward are that health care providers will see the need to evaluate the role that digital transformation has played on patient education and overall patient outcomes.

CLINICS CARE POINTS

- Clinicians are to know their audience when providing patient education.
- Select appropriate modalitiy for the patient education.
- Standardize the patient education using evidence based medical standards.
- Close follow up with patients that are struggling with access to and comprehension of technological advances in patient education.
- Assessment of patient education used by clinicians is should be the overall outcome of the patient's health and wellbeing.

DISCLOSURE

None.

REFERENCES

1. Stoumpos AI, Kitsios F, Talias MA. Digital transformation in healthcare: technology acceptance and its applications. Int J Environ Res Publ Health 2023;20(4). https://doi.org/10.3390/ijerph20043407.
2. May BJ. Patient Education Past and Present 1 (1). J Phys Ther Educ 1999; 13(3):3–7.
3. Chirumamilla S, Gulati M. Patient education and engagement through social media. Curr Cardiol Rev 2019;17(2):137–43.

4. de Mooij M, Foss O, Brost B. Integrating the experience: Principles for digital transformation across the patient journey. Digit Health 2022;8. https://doi.org/10.1177/20552076221089100.

5. Eriksen J, Bertelsen P, Bygholm A. The digital transformation of patient-reported outcomes' (PROS) functionality within healthcare. Stud Health Technol Inform 2020;270:1051–5.

6. de Mooij M, Foss O, Brost B. Integrating the experience: Principles for digital transformation across the patient journey. Digit Health 2022;8. 20552076221089100. Published 2022 Mar 30.

7. Eriksen J, Bertelsen P, Bygholm A. The digital transformation of patient-reported outcomes' (pros) functionality within healthcare. Stud Health Technol Inform 2020;270:1051–5.

8. Schooley B, Singh A, Hikmet N, et al. Integrated digital patient education at the bedside for patients with chronic conditions: observational study. JMIR Mhealth Uhealth 2020;8(12):e22947. PMID: 33350961; PMCID: PMC7785403.

9. Biblowitz K, Bellam S, Mosnaim G. Improving asthma outcomes in the digital era: a systematic review. Pharm Med 2018;32:173–87.

10. Golden AH, Gabriel MH, Russo J, et al. Let's talk about it: an exploration of the comparative use of three different digital platforms to gather patient-reported outcome measures. J Patient Rep Outcomes 2023;7:130.

11. Conard S. Best practices in digital health literacy. Int J Cardiol 2019;292:277–9.

12. Wonggom Parichat, Kourbelis Constance, Newman Peter, et al. Effectiveness of avatar-based technology in patient education for improving chronic disease knowledge and self-care behavior: a systematic review. JBI Database of Systematic Reviews and Implementation Reports 2019;17(6):1101–29.

13. Chandran VP, Balakrishnan A, Rashid M, et al. Mobile applications in medical education: A systematic review and meta-analysis. PLoS One 2022;17(3):e0265927. PMID: 35324994; PMCID: PMC8947018.

14. Morgan ER, Laing K, McCarthy J, et al. Using tablet-based technology in patient education about systemic therapy options for early-stage breast cancer: a pilot study. Curr Oncol 2015;22(5):364–9.

15. Poowuttikul P, Seth D. New concepts and technological resources in patient education and asthma self-management. Clin Rev Allergy Immunol 2020;59:19–37.

16. Shan R, Sarkar S, Martin SS. Digital health technology and mobile devices for the management of diabetes mellitus: state of the art. Diabetologia 2019;62:877–87.

17. Salim H, Cheong AT, Sharif-Ghazali S, et al. A self-management app to improve asthma control in adults with limited health literacy: a mixed-method feasibility study. BMC Med Inform Decis Mak 2023;23:194.

18. Guarnieri G, Caminati M, Achille A, et al. Severe asthma, telemedicine, and self-administered therapy: listening first to the patient. J Clin Med 2022;11(4):960.

19. Lombardo L, Wynne R, Hickman L, et al. New technologies call for new strategies for patient education. Eur J Cardiovasc Nurs 2021;20(5):399–401.

20. Morgan ER, Laing K, McCarthy J, et al. Using tablet-based technology in patient education about systemic therapy options for early-stage breast cancer: a pilot study. Curr Oncol 2015;22(5):364–9.

21. Al-Elq AH. Simulation-based medical teaching and learning. J Family Community Med 2010;17(1):35–40.

22. Pennecot C, Gagnayre R, Ammirati C, et al. Consensus Recommendations for the Use of Simulation in Therapeutic Patient Education. Simulat Healthc J Soc Med Simulat 2020;15(1):30–8.

23. van der Linde-van den Bor M, Slond F, Liesdek OCD, et al. The use of virtual reality in patient education related to medical somatic treatment: A scoping review. Patient Educ Couns 2022;105(7):1828–41.

24. Lin B, Wu S. Digital transformation in personalized medicine with artificial intelligence and the internet of medical things. OMICS 2022;26(2):77–81.

25. Dave M, Patel N. Artificial intelligence in healthcare and education. Br Dent J 2023;234(10):761–4.

26. Lawton G. What is generative ai? everything you need to know. 2023. Available at: https://cdn.ttgtmedia.com/rms/editorial/GenAI_Pillar_PDFdownload.pdf. [Accessed 28 December 2023].

27. Lahat A, Shachar E, Avidan B, et al. Evaluating the utility of a large language model in answering common patients' gastrointestinal health-related questions: are we there yet? Diagnostics 2023;13(11). https://doi.org/10.3390/diagnostics13111950.

28. Fujiwara Y, Nonaka K, Kuraoka M, et al. Influence of "face-to-face contact" and "non-face-to-face contact" on the subsequent decline in self-rated health and mental health status of young, middle-aged, and older japanese adults: a two-year prospective study. Int J Environ Res Publ Health 2022;19(4). https://doi.org/10.3390/ijerph19042218.

29. De Rezende LFM, Rey-López JP, Matsudo VKR, et al. Sedentary behavior and health outcomes among older adults: A systematic review. BMC Public Health 2014;14(1). https://doi.org/10.1186/1471-2458-14-333.

30. Gordon NP, Hornbrook MC. Older adults' readiness to engage with eHealth patient education and self-care resources: A cross-sectional survey. BMC Health Serv Res 2018;18(1). https://doi.org/10.1186/s12913-018-2986-0.

31. Curran VR, Hollett A, Peddle E. Patient Experiences with Virtual Care During the COVID-19 Pandemic: Phenomenological Focus Group Study. JMIR Form Res 2023;7. https://doi.org/10.2196/42966.

32. Batch BC, Spratt SE, Blalock DV, et al. General behavioral engagement and changes in clinical and cognitive outcomes of patients with type 2 diabetes using the time2focus mobile app for diabetes education: pilot evaluation. J Med Internet Res 2021;23(1). https://doi.org/10.2196/17537.

33. Thibault GE. The future of health professions education: Emerging trends in the United States. FASEB Bioadv 2020;2(12):685–94. PMID: 33336156; PMCID: PMC7734422.

Effective Communication Strategies for Patient Education

Kenneth E. Korber, PA, MHPE, DFAAPA

KEYWORDS

- Patient education ● Physician assistants ● Health literacy ● Effective communication
- Patient care ● Health care discussions

KEY POINTS

- Many Americans struggle to understand and use personal and public health information when it's filled with unfamiliar or complex terms.
- Effective communication between the physician assistants and the patient is a cornerstone of good health care.
- We can improve health literacy if we practice clear communication strategies and techniques. Clear communication means presenting familiar concepts, words, numbers, and images in ways that make sense to the people who need the information.
- Choosing to use jargon is an act of exclusion. Using clear communication advances health equity.
- Clear communication streamlines the translation process. That means you can more quickly share your information with people who are non-native English speakers and readers.

INTRODUCTION

As self-directed learners, physician assistants (PAs) are familiar with the notion that continuing professional development keeps us plugged into the advances of medicine and surgery and is part of our patient advocacy's "secret sauce." However, when it comes to our patient's perspective, they may not know what they don't know—despite patient education being part of our health advocacy goals. Therein lays a clinical challenge.

In this chapter, we explore the role of health literacy and special patient education situations where effective communication is tantamount to better health outcomes. You will learn how to adapt this knowledge to the continued success of your day-to-day patient care strategies.

Illinois Physician Assistant Training Program, Touro University & Health System, Skokie, IL 60076, USA
E-mail address: kenneth.korber@gmail.com

Physician Assist Clin 9 (2024) 479–486
https://doi.org/10.1016/j.cpha.2024.05.002   **physicianassistant.theclinics.com**
2405-7991/24/© 2024 Elsevier Inc. All rights are reserved, including those for text and data mining, AI training, and similar technologies.

Understanding Health Literacy

A person's literacy and health literacy are not the same but are related. Personal health literacy is the degree to which individuals can find, understand, and use information and services to inform health-related decisions and actions for themselves and others.

Health literacy is not a new phrase in organized medicine. Authors and researchers have written about general and health literacy for decades in the open-source literature.[1] The concept of health literacy evolved from a history of defining, redefining, and quantifying the functional literacy needs of the local adult population. Along with these changes has come the recognition that sophisticated literacy skills are increasingly needed to function in society and that low literacy may have a negative effect on health and health care delivery.

In early US history, definitions and measurement of literacy, in general, were crude. Before the Civil War, an individual's ability to sign his name on a legal document (rather than mark the document with an "X") was an indication of literacy.[2]

From the mid-1800s through the mid-1930s, the United States (US) Census Bureau merely asked individuals (initially white males) if they could read and write in any language. Using this approach, 20% of the population was deemed illiterate in the 1870s, but a century later (ie, 1979), only 0.6% of adults reported they could not read or write.[3] Though inexactly measured, this trend indicated that complete illiteracy became rare in the US.

In the twentieth century, more sophisticated definitions, conceptualizations, and measurements began to evolve in large part because military and labor experts were interested in determining what individuals needed to function on the job. The Civilian Conservation Corps coined the term "functional literacy" and defined it as having 3 or more years of schooling. For the next 30 years, literacy was defined in relation to increasing levels of school achievement, corresponding to the greater demands in the labor market and society overall. For example, in the 1940s, a fourth-grade education was considered the literacy level needed for various army jobs.[4]

By the 1950s, the US Census Bureau defined functional literacy as having at least a 6th-grade education. By the 1960s, as part of the War on Poverty, the Department of Education set a national standard of functional literacy as an 8th-grade education and expanded adult basic education programs to help achieve that goal.[5] This paradigm continued until the late 1970s, when it was thought that individuals needed at least a high school diploma to have an adequate level of general literacy.[3] Today, postsecondary training is often considered necessary for individuals to compete successfully in the labor market.

Public policy was influenced in the 1980s by the publication of "Toward a Literate Society," a report by reading researchers Carroll and Chall, which stated that, while illiteracy levels were declining, many individuals in the US continued to have severe reading problems.[6] Low literacy was identified as a national policy concern that would limit our economic, social, and defense competitiveness.[3,6]

The first major efforts to measure literacy in the adult population focused on real-world tasks but were limited to segments of the population. The Department of Education's 1985 National Assessment of Educational Progress tested young adults 21 to 25 years of age.[7]

Berkman and colleagues have documented the relationship between low literacy, health status, and health outcomes over the past 20 years.[8] This growing body of research has led to the formation of a new field of study: health literacy.

If you used "health literacy" as part of a contemporary PubMed citation database search, you would see that there has been an uptick in published citations related to this subject. In 2018, there were 2195 unique peer-reviewed articles published, and by the time 2022 came around, those article numbers reached 4074, an 86% increase. This surge in publications highlights the growing recognition of the importance of health literacy in health care research and practice.

Clinical Encounters

One corollary to successful patient education is the amount of engagement time we get to spend with our patients, whether in a hospital setting or through respective outpatient health systems.

In a recent 10-min online survey of US practicing physicians (n = 10,011), each was asked how much time was spent with patients within their respective work settings for the period of Oct 7, 2022, through Jan 17, 2023. In this report, we learned that most respondents spend no more than 20 minutes for each patient encounter. It, therefore, behooves us to develop a streamlined strategy to promote better understanding and "stickiness" to our prescribed teachable moments (eg, diagnostic workup progression, primary pharmacologic interventions, treatment monitoring and paths to an accurate prognosis).

Tailoring Communication to Different Age Groups

The linkage of health care delivery and health literacy in the US has evolved to include 3 additional patient education elements that enhance patient outcomes—Graph literacy, Numeracy literacy, and Picture Conversion techniques of verbal and written instructions. The following section parsed those education tools, based on the patient age category.

Adults

We all believe that good communication between the PA and the patient is a cornerstone of good health care. However, the reality is that a large number of adult patients cannot effectively participate in their own care because their literacy skills are subpar.[9] Compounding that challenge is the fact that clinicians use a specialized language ("medicalese") that may seem foreign to an outsider seeking care.

Low health literacy has also been highly correlated with excess hospitalizations.[10] This observation may suggest that an individual's decreased knowledge of self-care and reduced adherence contribute to a diminished ability to negotiate a complex health care system.

Clues that a patient may have inadequate health literacy include bringing a family member (which is good counsel anyway), wanting to discuss materials with a family member before adopting a shared decision-making strategy, claims of forgetting reading glasses, or incompletely or inadequately filling out forms in the practice or clinic. As mentioned above, patients may misunderstand many medical terms during any encounter. **Box 1** and **Table 1** outline strategies and examples for enhancing comprehension in adult patients with low health literacy.

Children

In the 2009 "Raising America" documentary, several startling revelations were presented to the television audience: (i) up to 20% of US kindergarten-aged children were not adequately prepared for the curricular and social assimilation process associated with that of an expected education journey into high school; (ii) neuroscience has demonstrated that a child's earliest surrounding and interactions shape the developing brain, building the foundations for lifelong cognitive and emotional development, even mental and physical health; and (iii) too often, families and communities are pressed by lack of time, money, and resources. These community factors feed

---

Box 1
Common recommendations for better oral exchange of information

- Ask patients how they learn best (reading, listening).

- Match teaching approaches to learning styles.

- Present a reasonable amount of information at one time.

- Avoid using organizational jargon or specialized words.

- Encourage questions.

- Assume the burden of clear communication by asking if the information or directions were clearly presented. For example, say, "Am I clear?" instead of, "Do you understand?"

- When appropriate, ask patients to repeat key points as though they were telling what they learned to a family member or friend. This approach enables the staff member to fill in missing information.

- Discuss key points of patient-centered videos (if materials were used in preparing a patient for a test or surgery).

Rudd RE, Anderson JE. The Health Literacy Environment of Hospitals and Health Centers. Partners for Action: Making Your Healthcare Facility Literacy-Friendly. 2006. www.hsph.harvard.edu/healthliteracy.[(p51)]

---

the trauma that adversely affects childhood experiences and facilitate outcomes that can get "under the skin" of young children—altering their brain architecture.[11] This powerful wake-up call should drive social justice campaigns, unleash better focus on the youngest members of society and contribute (directly) to the health literacy development of all children.

One innovative peer-to-peer resource was developed and presented as an oral poster at the 2019 Annual Academy of Physician Assistant annual CE|CME conference.[12]

Table 1
Improving understanding in a patient with low health literacy

What the Clinician Should Do	How to Achieve the Intended Results
Slow down	Take time to assess patients' literacy skills
Use "living room" language instead of reflex medical terminology	Use language that patients understand (including appropriate non-English language and not using 4-syllable words where simple words can explain the same message(s)
Show or draw pictures	Visual aids enhance understanding and subsequent recall
Limit information given at each patient encounter and repeat instructions. For pediatric patients, extend the encounter time with a bedtime reading tool.	
Use a "teach back" or "show me" approach to confirms patient's understanding	Ask patients to demonstrate their instructions to ensure that adequate instruction has been given. Never ask "Do you understand?" Typically, patients will say Yes even if they do not understand.
Be respectful, caring, and sensitive	An empathetic attitude reassures patients and helps them to improve participation in their own care.

The authors took the notion of a limited and time-restricted patient encounter environment and linked its health promotion messages to a familiar bedtime reading environment for pediatric patients. The material was also distributed to a select number of classrooms where reading circles were in place as facilitated reading skills events for emerging readers and other relevant learning environments, using the new character cohort and story narratives. One children's book was focused on the solution of tooth-brushing as a solution for better oral health, the second centered on salt substitution versus salty excess in diets of (targeting Hmong children at-risk for hypertension), another on a self-esteem challenge of children "feeling different" from other children, and the fourth provided engaging activities to drive home education of burn prevention and fire safety in the home for the youngest members of the family. In summary, the use of each published children's book title was engaging to these special pediatric populations, enhanced developmental discussion often experienced in a confusing outpatient setting, and provided reliable cartoon characters-as-teachers for emerging readers.[12]

Older adults
Navigation tools such as maps, signs, and staff are often available in health care facilities to help people find their way to and around the facility. However, these tools are only useful for patients when they are easily accessible and understandable.

Regarding the geriatric population, the telephone is often the first contact a person has with a health care facility. This initial interaction can shape a person's impressions of that health care facility.

An automated telephone system can be improved with the following adjustments.

1. Provide patients with the option to speak with a person.
2. Provide patients with the option to repeat menu items.
3. Use clear and simple language.
4. Use a conversational tone.
5. Use a slow speaking pace.
6. Provide patients with directions to the health care facility using multiple forms of transportation, including public transportation.

In addition, elderly patients are often inundated with materials (that the facility uses to focus on positive community relations, patient orientation, follow-up, patient education, legal materials, forms patients fill out, and discharge preparation information) when they go to a health care facility. These materials are only helpful for patients when they are written at the appropriate average reading grade level (~grade 8 or below) and have a simple layout and design.

Creating new materials [content]. When staff members develop new materials, they should consider the following key reminder: Use plain language. Plain language is defined as clear, simple, and conversational words and style. Plain language materials present information in a format that considers reading ease based on the organization and style of the text.

Creating new materials [design]. Care should also be centered on the print layout and design elements that make reading easy. The design of a material can make reading easier or more difficult. Recommendations can include the following:

Type and Spacing
1. Use a readable type style—a footed font (serif) in 12-point size.
2. Use appropriate spaces between lines—generally 1.2 to 1.5 spacing.

3. Provide good contrast between the paper and the text.
4. Do not print words on shaded or patterned background.
5. Use upper and lower case and avoid all CAPITAL LETTERS.
6. Include ample white space on the page.
Margins and Lines
1. Use large margins (at least 1 inch on each side).
2. Leave the right margin jagged (do not fully justify text).
3. Do not split words across 2 lines.

In the end, be consistent with patient-facing materials, avoid clutter on the page, provide a visual guide for finding key information, and clearly label all charts and illustrations. Nowadays, infographic designs are commonly used to convey important practice or care-related information.

Created material assessment. Many software tools (such as the SMOG, FRY, and the Flesch-Kincaid) are available to help assess the reading grade level of print materials. Most of these tools have been used extensively in education and have been well-tested. In addition, there are several tools available to help us conduct broader assessments of written health material. Each can be easily found via your preferred search engine or as part of a Microsoft Word document (pull-down menu in the review tab).

Clinically Sensitive Information/Tele-Communication

Remote monitoring, or telemonitoring, is becoming an increasingly popular alternative for maintaining surveillance of several medical conditions, including cancer.[13] Briefly, telemonitoring involves the transmission of relevant clinical information through digital means, which include internet-connected medical devices such as smartphones, health tracking apps, and video conferencing platforms. The main idea is to provide accurate and timely medical care, which can improve the patient's quality of life and reduce treatment costs by eliminating the need for regular in-person visits. This modality has given clinicians another tool in their patient management armamentarium, considering the significant epidemiologic importance of cancer for the population.

The use of telehealth has increased substantially in recent years, by more than 60-fold in 2020. Although telehealth made up less than 1% of medical visits before the coronavirus disease 2019 pandemic, it became ubiquitous with the onset of the pandemic, before tapering to still-unforeseen levels, with 37% of adults reporting at least 1 telephone or video visit in 2022.[14]

Shared Decision-Making

Shared decision-making is a collaboration in which the clinician explains treatment options, and the patient provides feedback on what they prefer. Shared decision-making is achieved when patients are empowered to be involved in all aspects of health care discussions and decision-making.[15]

Motivational Interviewing

Different strategies have been studied to enhance patient adherence to medications used for chronic illnesses.[16] Motivational interviewing (MI) is a patient-centered type of counseling that focuses on enhancing self-motivation and commitment to behavior change through collaborative and supportive communication with a health care provider.[16] MI-based interventions have demonstrated promising effects in improving medication adherence across a wide range of chronic conditions; including obesity and weight-loss management, the promotion of physical exercise, promoting oral hygiene, and informed consent related to vaccination in children. More recently, MI has been increasingly used in chronic condition management and especially in medication adherence for pain management settings.

Use of Interpreters

The Americans with Disabilities Act (ADA) requires that clinicians ensure effective communication with persons with disability, although it does not mandate specific communication modalities to achieve this goal. Instead, the ADA requires that patients' preferences be prioritized when choosing among communication options — such as American Sign Language (ASL) interpreters, communication access real-time translation, or auxiliary aids for persons with hearing deficits, and qualified readers, braille materials, and enlarged fonts for persons with low vision, 7 and various techniques for communicating with persons with intellectual disability.[17]

The 2011 World Report on Disability called for eliminating barriers to health care service delivery for persons with disability, including ensuring effective communication.[18] This was because clinicians frequently cite communication concerns as a challenge to providing high-quality health care. Recommendations for improving communication with people with disability included more ASL interpreters and accessible informational material (ie, placing responsibility for communication on the patient), such as arranging their own sign language interpreter to remove this responsibility from the respective practice.[19]

CLINICS CARE POINTS

- Typical challenging domains include: disease markers (eg, hemoglobin A1c, blood pressure, prostate specific antigen); functional capacity (eg, ability to walk); and communicating therapeutic regimens that lead to improved physical health (eg, medication, surgery, diet, smoking cessation and placebo effects).[20]

DISCLOSURE

The Author has nothing to disclose.

REFERENCES

1. Hedman-Robertson AS, Allison KG, Kerr DL, et al. Historical and contemporary aspects of health literacy in certified health education practice. Am J Health Educ 2021;52(6):323–32. https://doi.org/10.1080/19325037.2021.1976327.
2. Lockridge KA. Literacy in colonial New England: an inquiry into the social context of literacy in the early modern West. 1st edition. New York: W. W. Norton & Company; 1974.
3. Kaestle CF, Damon-Moore H, Stedman LC, et al. Literacy in the United States. New Haven (CT): Yale University Press; 1991.
4. Comings J, Kirsch I. Literacy skills of US adults. In: Schwartzberg JG, VanGeest JB, Wang CC, editors. Understanding health literacy: implications for medicine and public health. Chicago: American Medical Association Press; 2005. p. 43–53.
5. Kirsch I, Jungeblut A, Jenkins L, et al. Adult literacy in America: a first look at the results of the National Adult Literacy Survey. Washington, DC: National Center for Education Statistics, U.S. Department of Education; 1993.

6. Carroll JB, Chall JS. Toward a literate society. New York: McGraw-Hill; 1975.

7. Kirsch I, Jungeblut A. Literacy: profiles of America's young adults. Princeton (NJ): Educational Testing Service; 1986.

8. Berkman ND, DeWalt DA, Pignone MP, et al. Literacy and health outcomes. Evidence report/technology assessment No. 87 (AHRQ Publication No.04-E007-2). Rockville (MD): Agency for Healthcare Research and Quality; 2004.

9. Williams MV. Recognizing and overcoming inadequate health literacy: a barrier to care. Cleve Clin J Med 2002;69(5):415–8.

10. Baker DW, Parker RM, Williams MV, et al. Health literacy and the risk of hospitalization. J Gen Intern Med 1998;13:851–7.

11. The Raising of America – early childhood and the Future of our nation. The Raising of America | Documentary on the science of early childhood, working parents and public policy.

12. Korber KE, Possenti P. Qualitative assessment of Storybooks as Pt Ed Change-Makers. J Am Acad Physician Assistants 2019. https://doi.org/10.1097/01.jaa.0000603056.29644.74.

13. Martínez F, Tobar C, Taramasco C. Effects of internet-based telemonitoring platforms on the quality of life of oncologic patients: A systematic literature review protocol. PLoS One 2023;18(11):e0293948. PMID: 37939125; PMCID: PMC10631686.

14. Zhong A, Amat MJ, Anderson TS, et al. Completion of recommended tests and referrals in telehealth vs in-person visits. JAMA Netw Open 2023;6(11): e2343417. https://doi.org/10.1001/jamanetworkopen.2023.43417.

15. Yakubu RA, Coleman A, Ainyette A, et al. Shared decision-making and emergency department use among people with high blood pressure. Prev Chronic Dis 2023;20:E82. PMID: 37733952; PMCID: PMC10516202.

16. Papus M, Dima AL, Viprey M, et al. Motivational interviewing to support medication adherence in adults with chronic conditions: systematic review of randomized controlled trials. Patient Educ Counsel 2022;105:3186–203.

17. Agaronnik N, Campbell EG, Ressalam J, et al. Communicating with patients with disability: perspectives of practicing physicians. J Gen Intern Med 2019;34(7): 1139–45.

18. The World Report on Disability. Geneva: World Health Organization and The World Bank; 2011.

19. Roman G, Samar V, Ossip D, et al. Experiences of sign language interpreters and perspectives of interpreting administrators during the COVID-19 pandemic: a qualitative description. Publ Health Rep 2023;138(4):691–704. Epub 2023 May 27.

20. Rudd RE, Anderson JE. The Health Literacy Environment of Hospitals and Health Centers. Partners for Action: Making Your Healthcare Facility Literacy-Friendly. 2006. Available at: https://publications.worlded.org/WEIInternet/inc/common/_download_pub.cfm?id=16716&lid=3.

Empowering Patients Through Health Information

Jerica N. Derr, DMSc, PA-C[a,b,*], Katrina M. Schrode, PhD[c]

KEYWORDS

- Health literacy • Digital access • Patient empowerment • Evidence-based medicine

KEY POINTS

- Access to digital health information empowers patients to make informed decisions about their health and health care.
- The abundance of information available requires that patients be able to identify reliable information and avoid making decisions based on misinformation or conspiracy theories.
- Increased sharing of health information between organizations and with health trackers and apps requires careful consideration of privacy and security measures.
- Physician Assistants (PAs) and other providers should discuss these issues with their patients and implement workshops and trainings to facilitate their patients' health literacy for improved shared decision-making.

INTRODUCTION

In the digital age, the accessibility of health information has transformed health care, presenting both benefits and challenges. The ability to access reliable health data is crucial, enabling patients to make informed health decisions. However, the proliferation of online information necessitates sharp skills in discerning credible sources amid widespread misinformation and biased content. Misinformation, especially about sensitive topics like vaccination and weight management, poses significant hurdles, requiring health care providers to develop strategies to help patients evaluate and use evidence-based information effectively.

Additionally, the protection of health information privacy and security has become more critical than ever. The digital transformation in health data management demands stringent measures to prevent breaches and ensure ethical handling of sensitive information. This article explores how health care providers can enhance access

[a] Department of Physician Assistant Studies, A.T. Still University, Arizona School of Health Sciences, 5850 East Still Circle Mesa, Mesa, AZ 85206, USA; [b] Division of Physician Assistant Education, Oregon Health & Science University School of Medicine, Portland, Oregon, USA; [c] Department of Psychiatry, Charles R. Drew University of Medicine and Science, 1731 East 120th Street, Los Angeles, CA 90059, USA
* Corresponding author.
E-mail address: jericaderr@atsu.edu

Physician Assist Clin 9 (2024) 487–502
https://doi.org/10.1016/j.cpha.2024.05.003
physicianassistant.theclinics.com
2405-7991/24/© 2024 Elsevier Inc. All rights reserved, including those for text and data mining, AI training, and similar technologies.

to trustworthy health information and strategies for navigating online resources, debunking myths, and maintaining the confidentiality and security of personal health data. Embracing these essential aspects empowers patients to navigate the complexities of modern health care knowledgeably.

OBJECTIVES
Enhance Health Literacy and Digital Access

Boost health literacy and digital skills to enable effective use and understanding of online health information across different demographics.

Equip Patients with Skills to Evaluate Online Health Information

Provide educational tools to help patients critically assess online health content and distinguish credible sources from misinformation.Combat Misinformation and Conspiracy Theories

Formulate strategies to help patients recognize and refute health-related myths and conspiracy theories, especially concerning vaccines and weight management.

Ensure Health Information Privacy and Security

Implement protocols to protect patient privacy and secure health data online, while educating patients on safe digital practices for handling health information.

KEY CONCEPTS
Health Literacy

An individual's capacity to access, comprehend, and utilize health information to prevent disease, maintain health, and enhance quality of life.[1]

Digital Access

Access to reliable, high-speed internet enables accurate health information retrieval, telemedicine participation, and health monitoring technology use, but may be limited by costs, medical constraints, and digital complexity.[2]

Evidence-Based Medicine

Integrating data from clinical research with clinical expertise to optimize individual health care decisions.[3]

Patient Empowerment

When a patient can critically evaluate options and make informed autonomous health care decisions.[4]

BACKGROUND AND CONTEXT

The landscape regarding health information topics is continuously evolving due to technological advancements, societal changes, and ongoing efforts to address emerging challenges. Understanding the historical context is vital in devising effective strategies to address contemporary issues in health care information management.

Access to Reliable Health Information—Evolution of Information Dissemination

Historically, health information was accessed through printed materials, libraries, and health care professionals, with many also relying on non-official sources like friends, family, and cultural traditions. Advancements such as the printing press, public libraries, and educational campaigns gradually improved access. The emergence of the internet and digital technology revolutionized access to health information, offering vast resources but also posing challenges in quality control and credibility.[2]

The internet is a key source of health information through reputable websites, online portals, and apps, offering convenient access to extensive data. However, access disparities still affect underserved communities and those with limited digital literacy.[2] The vast amount of information also complicates distinguishing credible sources from misinformation.[5]

Evaluating Online Health Information

Rise of the Internet and Online Health Information: The internet dramatically changed how health information is accessed. Initially, health websites were few and generally trusted if they came from authoritative sources. As user-generated content and social media grew, discerning credible health information became more complex.[5] This shift from authoritative to user-generated content has changed how people judge information reliability.[6] The vast increase in online content has made assessing credibility tougher, with misinformation often spreading via social media.[5,6] Efforts to enhance digital health literacy, teaching people to critically evaluate and identify reliable sources, are ongoing.[7]

Misinformation and Conspiracy Theories

Historical Context of Medical Misinformation: Historically, health misinformation and conspiracy theories have shaped societal beliefs about treatments and illnesses, from ancient misconceptions to modern-day stigmas that deter some groups from accessing health care.[5,8] Events like the nineteenth-century anti-vaccine movement and misinformation during epidemics highlight the enduring influence of such beliefs on public health and policy.[9]

Today, health-related misinformation, especially regarding topics such as vaccines and weight management, proliferates across digital platforms.[10] False narratives, conspiracy theories, and misleading information contribute to hesitancy regarding scientifically proven treatments or preventive measures. Various entities, including health care professionals and social media platforms, are actively working to counter misinformation by debunking myths and promoting accurate information.[9,10]

Health Information Privacy and Security

Evolution of Data Protection and Privacy: Historically, patient information was stored in paper records and accessed by a few health care professionals. With the digitization of health records, concerns regarding privacy and security emerged.[11] Legislation like the Health Insurance Portability and Accountability Act (HIPAA) in the United States and the General Data Protection Regulation (GDPR) in Europe has evolved to address these issues.[11] The increasing use of health apps and wearable devices further underscores the need for robust security measures to protect personal health information and maintain privacy.[11]

THEORETIC FOUNDATIONS

The Health Belief Model (HBM) is a psychological framework designed to predict health behaviors by analyzing individuals' attitudes and beliefs toward health.[12] It consists of 6 key components that influence whether an individual is likely to adopt health-promoting behaviors. These include perceptions of severity, susceptibility, benefits of action, and barriers to action, self-efficacy, and cues to action.[12] The 6 components are described in **Table 1**.

Here are practical steps to effectively use the HBM in patient education.

Table 1	
The 6 key components of the Health Belief Model	
Perceived Susceptibility	Individuals' beliefs about their vulnerability to a particular health condition or illness. This component assesses the perceived risk of experiencing a health problem.
Perceived Severity	The perception of the seriousness or impact of a health problem if it occurs. It evaluates an individual's beliefs about the consequences, severity, or potential complications associated with the health issue.
Perceived Benefits	The beliefs regarding the effectiveness of taking a specific action to reduce the risk or seriousness of a health problem. This involves considering the advantages or positive outcomes linked to adopting recommended health behaviors.
Perceived Barriers	The perceived obstacles, challenges, or costs associated with performing a particular health behavior. This aspect assesses the potential hindrances or negative aspects that might deter an individual from adopting preventive actions.
Cues to Action	External or internal prompts that trigger the decision-making process regarding health behavior. These cues can be informational, environmental, or experiential, influencing an individual's readiness to take action.
Self-Efficacy	One's confidence in their ability to successfully execute and maintain a recommended health behavior. This component evaluates an individual's belief in their capacity to overcome obstacles and achieve the desired health outcome.

Assess Beliefs and Perceptions

Understand patients' views on their risk and the seriousness of health issues through surveys or discussions.

Tailor Information and Support

Provide personalized, evidence-based information that overcomes perceived barriers and highlights the benefits of positive behaviors. Offer guidance, encouragement, and resources to support patients in feeling capable of making health changes.

Engage and Follow Up

Maintain open communication, encourage participation, and prompt actions. Continuously follow up to reinforce behaviors, address concerns, and adjust educational approaches based on patient feedback and progress.

The Social Cognitive Theory (SCT), developed by Albert Bandura,[13] explains how individuals learn and adopt behaviors through observation, imitation, and interaction within social environments. SCT highlights the interplay between personal factors, behavior, and environment, stressing the importance of observational learning, self-regulation, self-efficacy, and environmental influences in behavior change and learning.[12,13] The key components of the SCT are outlined in **Table 2**.[13]

Here are some practical steps to apply SCT principles in patient education effectively.

Utilize Role Modeling

Conduct sessions where peers or experts demonstrate positive health behaviors and share success stories to inspire and instruct patients. These real-life examples can

Table 2
Key components of the Social Cognitive Theory

Observational Learning	Individuals learn behaviors by observing others, such as role models or peers, and the consequences of their actions. Observational learning involves paying attention to models, retaining the observed behaviors, and reproducing them when appropriate.
Behavioral Capability	Refers to an individual's knowledge and skillset to perform a particular behavior successfully. It involves the understanding and ability to execute the behavior when needed.
Expectations and Outcome Expectancies	Expectations regarding the consequences of a behavior influence whether an individual will engage in that behavior. Positive outcome expectancies (anticipating positive results) and negative outcome expectancies (anticipating negative consequences) impact behavioral choices.
Self-Efficacy	Central to social cognitive theory, self-efficacy refers to an individual's belief in their ability to successfully perform a specific behavior to achieve desired outcomes. Higher self-efficacy is associated with increased motivation and perseverance in behavior change efforts.
Self-Regulation and Goal Setting	Involves the process of setting goals, monitoring progress, and employing strategies to regulate and control behavior. Self-regulation includes self-monitoring, self-reflection, and self-reinforcement to achieve desired outcomes.
Environmental Factors	The social and physical environments influence behavior change. Factors such as social norms, support systems, access to resources, and reinforcement shape an individual's behavior and decision-making.
Reciprocal Determinism	The concept that behavior is influenced by a continuous interaction between personal factors, environmental factors, and behavior itself. These factors continuously interact and influence each other bidirectionally.
Modeling and Vicarious Learning	Individuals learn by observing and modeling the behaviors, attitudes, and emotional reactions of others. They can learn from both successful and unsuccessful models, shaping their behavior accordingly.
Outcome Expectations and Reinforcement	Individuals are motivated to perform behaviors based on the anticipated outcomes or reinforcements associated with those behaviors. Positive reinforcement increases the likelihood of repeating the behavior, while negative reinforcement reduces it.

serve as powerful models, inspiring patients and demonstrating the feasibility of behavior change.

Enhance Self-Efficacy

Assist patients in setting achievable goals and creating action plans. Offer workshops to develop practical skills such as reading nutrition labels or roleplay effective communication with health care providers, enhancing patients' confidence and abilities.

Create Supportive Environments

Direct patients to peer support groups and online communities. Use technology and social media to foster environments where patients can share experiences, receive support, and enhance their capacity for sustained behavior changes.

BEST PRACTICES AND STRATEGIES

The following are evidence-based strategies that can be used to improve health literacy, the ability to assess information quality, and facilitate shared decision-making. They implement concepts introduced by the HBM and SCT. The authors include examples of successful implementation.

Access to Reliable Health Information

Structured Health Literacy Programs: Providers should guide patients to online resources in clear language, preferably through their own websites or patient portals. For instance, Khan Academy[14] offers a comprehensive, free platform with reliable health information in its Health and Medicine section, which includes tutorials, articles, and videos on various medical topics. It is globally recognized and promotes health education and empowerment. Similarly, the National Institutes of Health provides a user-friendly portal with evidence-based resources for both patients and health care professionals, becoming a trusted source for credible medical insights[15] "Teach-backs," where patients repeat information back to the provider, effectively enhance health understanding.[16]

Additionally, structured patient education programs and workshops should be developed to boost health literacy, with materials to help patients access reliable health information and understand medical content.[7,17] Studies show that using digital evidence-based decision-making aids can increase perceived health literacy among patients faced with online health decisions.[17]

Evaluating Online Health Information

Critical Evaluation Training: Teach patients to identify reliable sources by checking for Health On the Net (HON) Code Certifications.[18] Websites with the HON seal adhere to stringent criteria for providing trustworthy health information. Direct patients to MedlinePlus, a comprehensive resource by the US National Library of Medicine, offering expert-curated information on a wide range of health topics including diseases, conditions, treatments, drugs, and wellness.[19] This platform is user-friendly and helps patients make informed health decisions.

Conduct critical evaluation training sessions to teach patients how to assess the credibility of online health resources.[20] Educate them on methods to evaluate website credibility and identify reliable sources.[20] Among individuals without a college degree, research by Kammerer and colleagues demonstrated that individuals with training in source evaluation were more effective in using objective information for decisions and felt more confident in their choices.[21] Enhancing critical evaluation skills, closely linked to health literacy, can improve patients' ability to discern reliable health information.[22]

Misinformation and Conspiracy Theories

Educational Campaigns and Materials: Conduct educational campaigns and create user-friendly materials to address health misinformation using evidence-based data and engaging formats.[9,17] For instance, during the COVID-19 pandemic, the Centers for Disease Control and Prevention in the United States launched a vaccine education initiative using their website, social media, and community programs to dispel myths and promote vaccination, which helped reduce vaccine hesitancy and build public trust.[23] Similarly, a coalition targeted misinformation in Hispanic communities by monitoring online Spanish conversations, using influencers in corrective campaigns, partnering with community organizations, and developing mass media communications to spread accurate information.[24] Physician Assistants (PAs), often at the forefront of patient-centered care, are well-placed to understand the roots of misinformation from interactions with patients, enabling them to lead efforts in correcting misconceptions. Additionally, websites like FactCheck.org rigorously analyze and debunk health myths, providing a valuable resource for evidence-based information.[25]

Health Information Privacy and Security

Privacy Awareness and Decision Support: Health data security is constantly evolving. For example, Guardtime uses cutting-edge blockchain technology to secure health data, ensuring tamper-proof records and safe data sharing.[26] Apple's Health Records feature allows users to securely store and access medical data on their devices, enhancing privacy and control over personal health information.[27] Providers can organize sessions to educate patients about health data privacy protections provided by companies like Guardtime and Apple, stressing the importance of informed consent.[28] Additionally, decision support tools and patient-centered communication techniques can be offered to actively involve patients in their care decisions.[28]

CLINICAL CARE POINTS

The following are tips for health care professionals and educators to successfully implement effective patient education practices.

I. *Tailored Information:* Adapt educational materials to meet the diverse needs of patients, considering their cultural backgrounds, literacy levels, and preferred languages.
II. *Use of Technology:* Implement user-friendly digital tools or apps that enhance access to reliable health information, provide evaluation features, and ensure privacy.
III. *Continuous Education:* Promote ongoing learning by keeping patients informed about new health information, technological updates, and changes in health care policies. Encourage open and non-judgmental responses to patient inquiries.

CHALLENGES AND CONSIDERATIONS

Empowering patients with accessible, reliable health information is vital for informed decision-making in health care. The digital age, however, brings challenges like disparities in accessing accurate information, evaluating vast online content, addressing misinformation, and ensuring data privacy and security. Cultural factors also significantly affect how diverse individuals use online health resources, react to misinformation, and view privacy concerns. Overcoming these barriers is critical to delivering customized information and promoting inclusivity, enabling all patients to make informed health decisions and engage actively in their care.

Access to Reliable Health Information

Patient access to reliable health information faces challenges from the digital divide and information overload.[29] Programs like the Obama Phone, Federal Communications Commission discounts, Veterans Pension, and Tribal Head Start program help low-income patients and vulnerable groups such as veterans and native Americans gain internet access.[30,31] However, those with digital access may struggle with the vast amount of online health information, finding it hard to identify trustworthy sources.[5,10] This issue is particularly acute for older adults and individuals with disabilities due to poor web accessibility, necessitating improvements like simplified language and better use of images.[32,33] Web accessibility of sites that contain health information remains low, resulting in diminished access for individuals with disabilities.[34] Improvements in accessibility in online information are necessary to facilitate access for these groups, including the use of images and plain language.[35] Providers sometimes worry that internet-informed patients might demand more time or rely on misinformation during consultations, limiting patient empowerment, but studies have shown that informed patients generally enhance care interactions.[36,37]

Ethical issues

Disparities in technology access create uneven opportunities for patient empowerment, raising ethical concerns about fairness in health care and worsening health inequalities, especially in marginalized and rural communities.[2,38–40]

Cultural and diversity considerations

Access and evaluation of online health information vary among cultural groups, with non-Hispanic white females more likely to seek such information than males or minorities.[41] First-generation migrants are also less likely to access information online.[42] Culturally tailored messages and multilingual resources can help bridge these gaps, promoting equitable access to health information for diverse populations.[43]

Evaluating Online Health Information

The ability of patients to critically evaluate online health information is crucial amidst widespread misinformation and digital illiteracy.[6,20] Many patients may opt for less reliable sources like social media due to limitations in health literacy, preferring these to recommended health care sources.[44,45] While videos on platforms like YouTube and TikTok can offer quality information, critical assessment is still necessary.[46,47] Despite the availability of workshops to enhance these skills, some patients may lack the capacity or willingness to participate, compounded by inadequate digital literacy.

Ethical issues

Disparities in the ability to critically assess health information create knowledge gaps that undermine patient empowerment and autonomy, particularly when misinformation influences decisions against established medical knowledge.[2,6] Commercial biases can also erode trust and informed decision-making. Moreover, stigma or personal beliefs may prevent providers from directing patients to evidence-based information, such as correcting misconceptions about human immunodeficiency virus (HIV), which is ethically problematic.[48]

Cultural and diversity considerations

Cultural beliefs significantly influence how individuals perceive and evaluate health information. Acknowledging these differences is vital for addressing biases and improving evaluation skills across diverse groups.[49] Culturally sensitive materials, tailored to align with various cultural contexts and dietary practices, ensure that health information is relevant and accessible, supporting effective communication and potentially motivating behavioral changes.[42,49,50] For example, tapping into certain cultural values such as religiosity or racial pride for African Americans or familialism for Latinos may be effective in motivating desired behavioral changes.[49]

Misinformation and Conspiracy Theories

Misinformation and conspiracy theories impact patient decision-making and emotional well-being, posing challenges in health care trust and engagement. Combating misinformation is difficult due to its prevalence and varied sources. It can be hard to change entrenched beliefs, especially those tied to religious or political identities.[44,51] Direct debunking may reinforce false beliefs, so providing correct information is a more effective strategy.[52]

In patient interactions, it is crucial to empower patients through shared decision-making. Initiating discussions about potential misinformation, listening to concerns, and empathizing are more effective than direct persuasion.[53,54] Building trust can guide patients toward credible sources and enhance health literacy, setting the stage for ongoing, preventive education against misinformation.[52]

Ethical issues

Misinformation, especially about critical health topics like vaccines or weight management, can undermine public health by promoting harmful practices and eroding trust in science-based health care.[52] This raises ethical concerns about autonomy and informed consent, particularly when patients make decisions based on flawed information. Ethical dilemmas intensify when conspiracy beliefs may impair decision-making capacity.[55]

Cultural and diversity considerations

Cultural beliefs often intersect with misinformation, particularly around historically sensitive topics such as mental and sexual health, influencing health decisions. Understanding cultural contexts influencing beliefs about health care can help address and correct misinformation effectively.[56] Addressing misinformation with cultural sensitivity is essential, acknowledging historical and systemic discrimination that may contribute to mistrust in government and health care entities.[56,57] Providers must respect diverse perspectives and avoid dismissing patient concerns as mere conspiracy theories. This approach, along with recognizing that different cultures may prefer different online information sources, helps tailor effective interventions.[58]

Health Information Privacy and Security

The digitalization of health records has raised concerns about data breaches and transparency in patient privacy.[11] Many patients are not fully aware, or may not even care, how their health information is managed, used, or shared, particularly with the use of wearable devices and mobile health apps.[59–61] This lack of transparency can deter patients from engaging with online health resources and affect their trust and empowerment in the health care system.[61] Providers should ensure that patients are aware of the importance of safeguarding their health information.

Ethical considerations

Maintaining confidentiality and trust in the management of health information is ethically crucial. Breaches or inadequate data security jeopardize patient trust and raise ethical concerns about the handling of sensitive data. Ensuring patients have control over their health data and informed consent for its use is paramount.[62] Devices and apps that fail to ensure secure data handling or consent processes violate ethical standards.[60]

Cultural and diversity considerations

Cultural attitudes toward privacy vary and influence perceptions of health information security. It is important to respect these norms to build trust and ensure effective communication with diverse populations. Some groups, like refugees or undocumented migrants, may be particularly cautious about sharing health information due to fears of data reaching unintended parties.[63] Addressing these concerns with culturally sensitive data security measures is essential for fostering patient empowerment and trust.

FUTURE DIRECTIONS AND OPPORTUNITIES

The health care information landscape is rapidly evolving, propelled by trends that boost patient empowerment. Notable advancements such as telehealth expansion, artificial intelligence (AI) in health assistance, collaborative fact-checking platforms, and enhanced data protection are enhancing access to accurate information, combating misinformation, and reinforcing privacy. These developments are shaping a future where technology and strategic improvements support informed decision-making and equitable health care access, with ongoing research aimed at further progress.

Emerging Trends

Access to reliable health information
Telehealth services boost access to reliable health information through remote consultations, medical records access, and health education, overcoming geographic barriers.[40] AI tools and chatbots further enhance this by providing personalized health navigation and immediate responses.[64]

Evaluating online health information
New apps improve health literacy by helping users evaluate online health information with guidance, fact-checking, and evaluation tools.[65] Blockchain technology is also used to verify the authenticity of sources, enhancing transparency and credibility.[11]

Misinformation and conspiracy theories
Collaborative efforts among health care professionals, fact-checkers, and social media platforms aim to counter misinformation.[52,56] These initiatives use multimedia, storytelling, and user-generated content to debunk false claims and promote accurate information, encouraging healthier behaviors.[52]

Health information privacy and security
Regulations like GDPR enhance data protection, ensuring patients' rights to privacy and security.[11] Blockchain technology is increasingly used in health care for secure data exchange and maintaining patient consent, boosting trust in health information systems.[11,62]

Recommendations

Access to reliable health information
Mobile Health (mHealth) platforms, wearables, and apps broaden access to health information, offering educational resources, remote consultations, and health-tracking tools that engage and empower patients, especially those in remote or underserved areas.[11] Future improvements should focus on user-friendliness and integration with health records. Collaborative community-based efforts with health workers and organizations also enhance access by providing locally tailored information.[17,56] Ongoing research is necessary to evaluate the effectiveness and user acceptance of mHealth tools across diverse populations.

Evaluating online health information
Health care professionals guide patients in navigating online health resources.[20] While evidence on the effectiveness of interventions to improve online health literacy is limited, future research should involve large, diverse studies.[66] Chatbots have shown

potential for providing easy access to reliable health information, but must be regularly updated and designed inclusively with data from underrepresented groups to avoid biases.[67,68]

Misinformation and conspiracy theories

Public health campaigns that debunk myths and conspiracy theories about topics like vaccines and weight management are crucial. Such campaigns can include clinic-based video clips, direct mailings, and community-led discussions, leveraging peer influence for greater impact.[69,70] Integrating health and media literacy into education further empowers individuals to critically assess information and make informed decisions.[53]

Health information privacy and security

Tools and platforms that let patients manage their health data promote empowerment and strengthen autonomy and trust in health care.[7,71] Secure patient portals and consent processes are essential, especially as precision medicine and predictive algorithms become more prevalent.[62] These technologies must protect patient data rigorously and be developed inclusively to ensure their effectiveness and fairness across all patient groups.[68,72]

SUMMARY

In today's digital age, the vast availability of health information online can empower patients by enhancing their understanding of preventative and chronic health care, thereby improving decision-making and patient-provider collaboration. However, boosting health literacy is essential so patients can discern reliable, evidence-based information from misinformation and conspiracy theories. As health data increasingly circulates between organizations and mHealth devices, patients must also learn to safeguard their personal information. Despite the general availability of online health resources, disparities remain in access and the ability to critically assess this information. Health care providers should guide patients toward trustworthy sources, expect and address misinformation, and foster an open dialogue. By treating patients with patience and respect, providers can encourage critical thinking and informed health decisions.

CLINICS CARE POINTS

- Empowering Patient-Centered Care: Encourage patients to actively participate in their healthcare decisions by providing personalized health education and facilitating open discussions about their preferences and concerns.

- Addressing Digital Literacy: Offer workshops and resources to improve patients' digital literacy, enabling them to navigate and use digital health tools effectively, which can enhance their overall healthcare experience.

- Cultural Competency in Health Education: Develop culturally tailored educational materials and programs that consider the unique beliefs, values, and health practices of diverse patient populations to ensure inclusivity and effectiveness.

- Interactive Learning Tools: Utilize interactive digital tools such as apps and online modules that provide engaging, evidence-based health information, helping patients understand complex medical concepts and make informed decisions.

- Ongoing Patient Support: Implement regular follow-up sessions to reinforce health education, address any misconceptions, and provide continuous support for patients in managing their health conditions.

- Privacy Education: Educate patients about the importance of protecting their health information, including the use of secure passwords, recognizing phishing attempts, and understanding privacy settings on health apps and devices.
- Integration of Technology in Care: Incorporate telehealth and remote monitoring technologies into patient care plans, ensuring that patients are comfortable and proficient in using these tools for better health outcomes.
- Critical Thinking and Evaluation: Teach patients critical thinking skills to evaluate the reliability of online health information, encouraging them to consult reputable sources and healthcare providers for verification.
- Community Engagement: Engage with community organizations to disseminate health information and resources, leveraging local networks to reach underserved populations and improve health literacy.
- Feedback Mechanisms: Establish feedback mechanisms such as surveys and suggestion boxes to gather patient input on educational materials and programs, ensuring they meet the evolving needs of the patient population.

DISCLOSURE

The authors declare that they have no commercial or financial conflicts of interest in relation to the research detailed in this article. Additionally, they affirm that there are no external funding sources to disclose.

REFERENCES

1. Sørensen K, Van den Broucke S, Fullam J, et al. Health literacy and public health: a systematic review and integration of definitions and models. BMC Public Health 2012;12:1–13.
2. Estacio EV, Whittle R, Protheroe J. The digital divide: examining socio-demographic factors associated with health literacy, access and use of internet to seek health information. J Health Psychol 2019;24(12):1668–75.
3. Sackett DL, Rosenberg WM, Gray JA, et al. Evidence based medicine: what it is and what it isn't. BMJ 1996;312(7023):71–2.
4. Anderson RM, Funnell MM. Patient empowerment: myths and misconceptions. Patient Educ Couns 2010;79(3):277–82.
5. Grimes DR. Health disinformation & social media: The crucial role of information hygiene in mitigating conspiracy theory and infodemics. EMBO Rep 2020;21(11):e51819.
6. Petersen A, Tanner C, Munsie M. Navigating the cartographies of trust: how patients and carers establish the credibility of online treatment claims. Sociol Health Illn 2019;41(S1):50–64.
7. Cheng C, Gearon E, Hawkins M, et al. Digital health literacy as a predictor of awareness, engagement, and use of a National Web-Based Personal Health Record: population-based survey study. J Med Internet Res 2022;24(9):e35772.
8. Curtis MG, Whalen CC, Pjesivac I, et al. Contextual pathways linking cumulative experiences of racial discrimination to black american men's COVID Vaccine Hesitancy. J Racial Ethn Health Disparities 2022;1–13.
9. Enders AM, Uscinski J, Klofstad C, et al. On the relationship between conspiracy theory beliefs, misinformation, and vaccine hesitancy. PLoS One 2022;17(10):e0276082.
10. Germani F, Pattison AB, Reinfelde M. WHO and digital agencies: how to effectively tackle COVID-19 misinformation online. BMJ Glob Health 2022;7(8):e009483.

11. Jennath HS, Anoop VS, Asharaf S. Blockchain for healthcare: securing patient data and enabling trusted artificial intelligence. International journal of interactive multimedia and artificial intelligence 2020;6(3):15–23.
12. Sharma M. Theoretical Foundations of Health Education and Health Promotion. Third edition. Burlington, MA: Jones & Bartlett Learning; 2017.
13. Bandura A, Kazdin AE. Encyclopedia of Psychology, vol. 7. New York, NY, Washington: Oxford University Press; 2000. p. 329–32.
14. Health and medicine | Science. Available at: https://www.khanacademy.org/science/health-and-medicine. [Accessed 17 December 2023].
15. Health information. Available at: https://www.nih.gov/health-information. [Accessed 17 December 2023].
16. Yen PH, Leasure AR. Use and effectiveness of the teach-back method in patient education and health outcomes. Fed Pract 2019;36(6):284.
17. Wehkamp K, Kiefer FB, Geiger F, et al. Enhancing specific health literacy with a digital evidence-based patient decision aid for hypertension: a randomized controlled trial. Patient Prefer Adherence 2021;1269–79.
18. Health On the Net Foundation (HON). Available at: https://imia-medinfo.org/wp/health-on-the-net-foundation-hon. [Accessed 17 December 2023].
19. MedlinePlus - health information from the National Library of Medicine. Available at: https://medlineplus.gov/. [Accessed 17 December 2023].
20. Chiu Y-L, Tsai C-C, Liang J-C. Laypeople's online health information search strategies and use for health-related problems: cross-sectional survey. J Med Internet Res 2022;24(9):e29609.
21. Kammerer Y, Amann DG, Gerjets P. When adults without university education search the Internet for health information: The roles of Internet-specific epistemic beliefs and a source evaluation intervention. Comput Human Behav 2015;48:297–309.
22. Diviani N, van den Putte B, Giani S, et al. Low health literacy and evaluation of online health information: a systematic review of the literature. J Med Internet Res 2015;17(5):e112.
23. Education info about vaccines and diseases they prevent | CDC. Updated 2023-11-01T01:11:08Z. Accessed Web Page, 2023. Available at: https://www.cdc.gov/vaccines/ed/patient-ed.html.
24. Silesky MD, Panchal D, Fields M, et al. A multifaceted campaign to combat COVID-19 misinformation in the hispanic community. J Community Health 2023;48(2):286–94.
25. Health archives. Available at: https://www.factcheck.org/issue/health/. [Accessed 17 December 2023].
26. Guardtime health — guardtime. Available at: https://guardtime.com/health. [Accessed 17 December 2023].
27. Healthcare - health records. Available at: https://www.apple.com/healthcare/health-records/. [Accessed 17 December 2023].
28. Siebinga VY, Driever EM, Stiggelbout AM, et al. Shared decision making, patient-centered communication and patient satisfaction – A cross-sectional analysis. Patient Educ Couns 2022;105(7):2145–50.
29. Powell J, Deetjen U. Characterizing the digital health citizen: mixed-methods study deriving a new typology. J Med Internet Res 2019;21(3):e11279.
30. Obama phone program. Available at: https://www.obamaphone.com/. [Accessed 17 December 2023].
31. Affordable connectivity program. Available at: https://www.fcc.gov/acp. [Accessed 17 December 2023].

32. Agree EM, King AC, Castro CM, et al. "It's got to be on this page": Age and cognitive style in a study of online health information seeking. J Med Internet Res 2015; 17(3):e3352.

33. Robinson L, Schulz J, Blank G, et al. Digital inequalities 2.0: Legacy inequalities in the information age. Clin Hemorheol Microcirc 2020;25(7).

34. Mason AM, Compton J, Bhati S. Disabilities and the digital divide: assessing web accessibility, readability, and mobility of popular health websites. J Health Commun 2021;26(10):667–74.

35. Terras MM, Jarrett D, McGregor SA. The importance of accessible information in promoting the inclusion of people with an intellectual disability. Disabilities 2021; 1(3):132–50.

36. Masters K, Ng'ambi D, Todd G. "I Found it on the Internet": Preparing for the e-patient in Oman. Sultan Qaboos Univ Med J 2010;10(2):169.

37. Ferguson T. Online patient-helpers and physicians working together: a new partnership for high quality health care. BMJ 2000;321(7269):1129–32.

38. Chen X, Orom H, Hay JL, et al. Differences in rural and urban health information access and use. J Rural Health 2019;35(3):405–17.

39. Lee JG, LePrevost CE, Harwell EL, et al. Coronavirus pandemic highlights critical gaps in rural Internet access for migrant and seasonal farmworkers: a call for partnership with medical libraries. J Med Libr Assoc 2020;108(4):651.

40. Al Haque E, Smith AD, Johnson B. Towards equitable healthcare: a cross dataset analysis of healthcare and telehealth access. Proceedings of the Association for Information Science and Technology 2023;60(1):11–20.

41. Din HN, McDaniels-Davidson C, Nodora J, et al. Profiles of a health information-seeking population and the current digital divide: Cross-sectional analysis of the 2015-2016 California health interview survey. J Med Internet Res 2019;21(5): e11931.

42. Samkange-Zeeb F, Borisova L, Padilla B, et al. Superdiversity, migration and use of internet-based health information–results of a cross-sectional survey conducted in 4 European countries. BMC Public Health 2020;20:1–12.

43. Alsan M, Stanford FC, Banerjee A, et al. Comparison of knowledge and information-seeking behavior after general COVID-19 public health messages and messages tailored for Black and Latinx communities: a randomized controlled trial. Annals of internal medicine 2021;174(4):484–92.

44. Featherstone JD, Bell RA, Ruiz JB. Relationship of people's sources of health information and political ideology with acceptance of conspiratorial beliefs about vaccines. Vaccine 2019;37(23):2993–7.

45. Von Wagner C, Semmler C, Good A, et al. Health literacy and self-efficacy for participating in colorectal cancer screening: the role of information processing. Patient Educ Couns 2009;75(3):352–7.

46. Song S, Xue X, Zhao YC, et al. Short-video apps as a health information source for chronic obstructive pulmonary disease: information quality assessment of TikTok videos. J Med Internet Res 2021;23(12):e28318.

47. Valera P, Acuna N, Alzate-Duque L, et al. The development and prototype feedback of digital cancer 101 videos to enhance cancer education for marginalized communities with limited health literacy. Cancer Control 2021;28. 10732748211006055.

48. Calabrese SK, Mayer KH, Marcus JL. Prioritising pleasure and correcting misinformation in the era of U= U. The Lancet HIV 2021;8(3):e175–80.

49. Tan NQ, Cho H. Cultural appropriateness in health communication: a review and a revised framework. J Health Commun 2019;24(5):492–502.

50. Duffy L, Burt KG. Exploring the relationship between cultural humility and professional diversity through the biased mediterranean diet. J Best Pract Health Prof Divers 2020;13(2):174–83.

51. Ecker UK, Lewandowsky S, Cook J, et al. The psychological drivers of misinformation belief and its resistance to correction. Nature Reviews Psychology 2022; 1(1):13–29.

52. Roozenbeek J, Van Der Linden S. How to combat health misinformation: a psychological approach. Los Angeles, CA: SAGE Publications Sage; 2022. p. 569–75.

53. Schulz PJ, Nakamoto K. The perils of misinformation: when health literacy goes awry. Nat Rev Nephrol 2022;18(3):135–6.

54. Southwell BG, Niederdeppe J, Cappella JN, et al. Misinformation as a misunderstood challenge to public health. Am J Prev Med 2019;57(2):282–5.

55. Stout N. Conspiracy theories and clinical decision-making. Bioethics 2023. https://doi.org/10.1111/bioe.13146.

56. Okoro O, Kennedy J, Simmons G, et al. Exploring the scope and dimensions of vaccine hesitancy and resistance to enhance COVID-19 vaccination in black communities. Cham: Springer International Publishing; 2022. p. 2117–30.

57. Jaiswal J, LoSchiavo C, Perlman DC. Disinformation, misinformation and inequality-driven mistrust in the time of COVID-19: lessons unlearned from AIDS denialism. AIDS Behav 2020;24(10):2776–80.

58. Chong SK, Ali SH, Đoàn LN, et al. Social media use and misinformation among Asian Americans during COVID-19. Front Public Health 2022;9:764681.

59. Cilliers L. Wearable devices in healthcare: Privacy and information security issues. Health Inf Manag J 2020;49(2–3):150–6.

60. Alfawzan N, Christen M, Spitale G, et al. Privacy, data sharing, and data security policies of women's mhealth apps: scoping review and content analysis. JMIR Mhealth and Uhealth 2022;10(5):e33735.

61. Shen N, Sequeira L, Silver MP, et al. Patient privacy perspectives on health information exchange in a mental health context: qualitative study. JMIR Mhealth 2019;6(11):e13306.

62. Spanakis EG, Sfakianakis S, Bonomi S, et al. Emerging and established trends to support secure health information exchange. Frontiers in Digital Health 2021;3: 636082.

63. Deal A, Hayward SE, Huda M, et al. Strategies and action points to ensure equitable uptake of COVID-19 vaccinations: a national qualitative interview study to explore the views of undocumented migrants, asylum seekers, and refugees. J Migr Health 2021;4:100050.

64. Liu T, Xiao X. A Framework of AI-based approaches to improving ehealth literacy and combating infodemic. Front Public Health 2021;9:755808.

65. Göransson C, Wengström Y, Hälleberg-Nyman M, et al. An app for supporting older people receiving home care - usage, aspects of health and health literacy: a quasi-experimental study. BMC Med Inform Decis Mak 2020;20(1):226.

66. Car J, Lang B, Colledge A, et al. Interventions for enhancing consumers' online health literacy. Cochrane Database Syst Rev 2011;6. https://doi.org/10.1002/14651858.cd007092.pub2.

67. Xiao Z, Liao QV, Zhou M, et al. Powering an AI chatbot with expert sourcing to support credible health information access. Sydney, NSW, Australia: presented at: Proceedings of the 28th International Conference on Intelligent User Interfaces; 2023. https://doi.org/10.1145/3581641.3584031.

68. Cahan EM, Hernandez-Boussard T, Thadaney-Israni S, et al. Putting the data before the algorithm in big data addressing personalized healthcare. NPJ Digital Medicine 2019/08/19 2019;2(1):78.

69. Ugarte DA, Young S. Effects of an online community peer-support intervention on COVID-19 vaccine misinformation among essential workers: mixed-methods analysis. West J Emerg Med 2023;24(2):264.

70. Sundstrom B, Cartmell KB, White AA, et al. Correcting HPV vaccination misinformation online: Evaluating the HPV vaccination NOW social media campaign. Vaccine 2021;9(4):352.

71. Alipour J, Mehdipour Y, Karimi A, et al. Security, confidentiality, privacy and patient safety in the hospital information systems from the users' perspective: a cross-sectional study. Int J Med Inf 2023;175:105066.

72. Thapa C, Camtepe S. Precision health data: Requirements, challenges and existing techniques for data security and privacy. Comput Biol Med 2021;129:104130.

Team-Based Approach to Patient Education

Sampath Wijesinghe, DHSc, MS, MPAS, PA-C, AAHIVS[a],
Brent Luu, PharmD, BCACP[b],*, Teuta Kadiu, RN, PhD[b]

KEYWORDS

- Healthcare literacy • Team-based approach to patient education
- Collaborative practice • Collaboration • Partnership

KEY POINTS

- Patients' outcomes may be significantly improved by team-based approach (TBA) to patient education.
- While prioritizing and implementing TBA to patient education, there are several critical considerations that need to be assessed and defined. These include role clarification, communication infrastructure, shared space for collaboration, team-based trust, and organizational support.
- Current systematic review suggests creating more opportunities for TBA in patient education, standardized patient education resources, a team-based education, a leadership role education, and a team-based quality improvement training program.

INTRODUCTION

Patient education plays a crucial role in healthcare, impacting patient safety and outcomes. To enhance its effectiveness, a team-based approach (TBA) is recommended due to the growing complexity of the healthcare system. Disease management often necessitates collaborative efforts, emphasizing the importance of teamwork in achieving optimal patient education. This collaboration, known as interprofessional collaboration (IPC), involves professionals from different disciplines working together to deliver services beyond individual capabilities.[1] Successful IPC in healthcare requires clinical expertise, effective communication, and a positive attitude. A supportive culture, whether within or across professions and groups, fosters IPC. In healthcare settings, IPC manifests as a TBA where professionals with distinct roles collaborate to enhance processes and achieve better patient outcomes. Unlike

[a] School of Medicine, Stanford University, 1265 Welch Road, Suite 100, Stanford, CA 94305, USA; [b] Betty Irene Moore School of Nursing, UC Davis, 2570 48th Street, Sacramento, CA 9587, USA
* Corresponding author. Betty Irene Moore School of Nursing, 2570 48th Street, Sacramento, CA 9587.
E-mail address: brluu@ucdavis.edu

Physician Assist Clin 9 (2024) 503–513
https://doi.org/10.1016/j.cpha.2024.05.004
2405-7991/24/© 2024 Elsevier Inc. All rights reserved, including those for text and data mining, AI training, and similar technologies.

IPC, which relies on shared values, teams are structured with defined roles and responsibilities. Institutions can promote IPC by establishing structures that facilitate team-based patient care. For example, a specific team could consist of healthcare professionals from various medical specialties and primary care providers (PCPs). Alternatively, the team might include physician associates, physicians, nurses, social workers, and pharmacists, all customized to address the requirements of the patient demographic. The implementation of IPC via such teams has been associated with enhanced patient outcomes, encompassing satisfaction, education, and medication adherence.[1,2]

In the early 1990s, about half of all premature deaths in the United States (US) were due to factors like low physical activity, smoking, and unhealthy diets.[3] A study from 2009, which involved over 23,000 participants, found that those who followed 4 healthy habits—like not smoking, maintaining a body mass index under 30, being physically active, and eating healthily—had a 78% lower risk of chronic diseases such as diabetes, heart attacks, strokes, and cancer compared to those who did not follow any of these habits.[4] These chronic diseases, largely influenced by human behavior, can be significantly reduced or prevented through patient education. Essentially, adopting healthy behaviors can greatly reduce the likelihood of developing these diseases, and patient education plays a crucial role in achieving this. Additionally, patients are often eager to learn more about their medical conditions, including general aspects of their illness, proper medication usage, and potential interactions with other drugs or foods to avoid complications. To build any necessary intentional redundancy and enhance the consistency, as well as the diversity of the provided educational information to patients, in this article, the authors will explore different paradigms of the TBA to patient education and their challenges.

BACKGROUND

The TBA to patient education requires the collaboration of different professionals. This IPC within healthcare system has been suggested and implemented for many years due to the observed improvement of patient outcomes such as reduction of preventable adverse drug reactions, increased therapeutic optimization, or decreased morbidity and mortality.[3] Additionally, TBA has also led to reduction of extrawork from healthcare professionals, therefore, greater job satisfaction.[4] Together with the current availability of technologies such as mobile devices, laptops, and social media, they have brought the collaboration between different disciplines even closer.[5,6] The pressure of the coronavirus disease 2019 (COVID-19) pandemic has pushed many sectors of healthcare, if not all, to online meeting platforms such as Zoom, Webex, or Teams, which could further and conveniently facilitate the participation of any discipline broadly across a large geographic areas, which may be historically limited. The key concepts of relevant collaboration has been reviewed and reported previously, which may include 5 different elements, namely *sharing, partnership, interdependency, power,* and *process.*[7] Under the *sharing* category, it may include shared values, shared responsibilities, shared philosophies, shared data, shared planning and interventions, shared professional perspectives, or shared decision-making.[7] From this spirit of sharing, it leads to the notion of *partnership*, which is a collegial relationship between 2 or more parties who are willing to collaborate. The core structure of *partnership* must be based on an opened and transparent bidirectional communication, which is then nurtured by mutual trust and respect, to achieve the common goals. Once the partnership has developed and matured, each party involved in the collaboration is interdependent on each other to address the needs of patients. This interdependency is heavily reliant on the expertise and contributions of the participants or the healthcare professionals. When all members of the team have realized the expertise and interdependency amongst the members, the inputting efforts will be synergistically amplified and resulted in more impactful outcomes.[7] The concept of empowerment of each party within the circle of IPC is much needed because it is the shared power among the team members that will bring and enhance relationship, which is based on experience and knowledge rather than titles or functions.[7] Lastly, collaboration could also be accepted as an evolving *process*, which may be interactive and dynamic, or transformative and interpersonal. This process may involve phases of negotiation and compromise while making decisions in planning or intervention. Furthermore, it may also involve steps that transcended the professional restrictions of each team member with the given satisfactory professional skills and qualities if the contribution is to better patient outcomes.[7] This model of IPC may be summarized in **Fig. 1**.

According to a literature review in 2005, there were several theoretic frameworks of collaboration, which were derived from the organizational theory; the organizational sociology theory; the social exchange theory; and other mixed frameworks, because collaboration does not necessarily occur by simply bringing professionals together in a team.[7] Under the organizational theory, the model proposed the inputs as group composition, cultural and organizational context, and the involving tasks. Meanwhile, the variables that influence the effectiveness of the collaboration included leadership, decision-making, and communication. Lastly, the outputs referred to performance, well-being, viability, and innovation of the team. This model has been used to study many national health systems in the United Kingdom.[7] On the other hand, the organizational sociology theory conceptualizes the collaboration process according to 4 elements: (a) shared goals and vision (ie, refers as finalization); (b) a sense of belonging (ie, interiorization); (c) strengthening structures by defining structural rules to regulate action (ie, formalization); and (d) governance (ie, central or local leadership, expertise and connectivity).[7] Additionally, under the social exchange theory, collaboration may be understood through interpersonal transactions, which consist of exchange and negotiation. For example, an individual joins a team that provides a specific benefit; in exchange he must help the team to realize its objectives. In parallel, the negotiation begins when the person offers to contribute his specific expertise to the team and in return expects to receive the specific benefits. From the analysis of these theoretic frameworks of collaboration, this study revealed that collaborative processes are derived from the 2 goals: (a) to serve the client needs; and (b) to serve the professional needs. As a result, the key elements of collaboration may be defined by (1) constructing a collective action that addresses the complexity of client's needs, and (2) constructing a team that integrates the perspectives of each member and fosters respect and trust for each other.[7] In general, IPC practice could be organized into 3 different elements, in which collaboration consists of inputs, processes, and outputs, where outputs are the efficiency

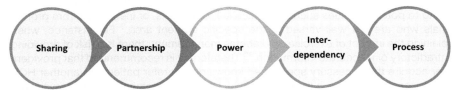

Fig. 1. The key relevant elements of interprofessional collaboration.

of the team, and inputs are the professional, organizational, or structural factors that affect the process.[7]

BARRIERS AND CHALLENGES WHILE IMPLEMENTING TEAM-BASED APPROACH TO PATIENT EDUCATION

When TBA is implemented during patient education, clinicians may encounter a variety of potential barriers that occur within the environment of IPC. For instance, the transition from non-IPC to IPC–that is, what are the signals or precipitating events in the systems prior to the onset of collaboration, and when does a collaborator know that its work is done. Other barriers to IPC may occur due to conflict interactions between individuals, collaborative team, and the organization. A provider, for example, may have different values and goals from those of the entire collaborative team. Indeed, he or she may be tasked to attend to the needs of larger number of patients and families, which may limit participation and communication with other members of the team. Limited participation and communication can negatively impact the performance and outcomes of the target system, deteriorate trust within the team and lead to provider burnout. Wei and colleagues reported "role clarity" as a barrier to IPC.[8] However, a possible solution to managing the conflicting demands from various entities within a collaborative team may need a collective skillfulness of sharing the responsibility of problem-solving in the best interests of the patients and the caregivers by paying attention to the other professional jurisdiction in addition to their own. In addition, challenges such as the lack of time among healthcare providers (HCPs), insufficient specialized knowledge, limited IPC, redundant education by different providers, inconsistent education practices, high provider turnover, dependence on Electronic Medical Records (EMR) for patient education, and challenges linked to patients may also involve during the TBA to patient education.

Lack of Time

The time constraints faced by HCPs present a significant obstacle to patient education. Providers often struggle with limited time for personalized or recurring education sessions with patients.[9,10] This lack of time emerges as a major barrier to effective education. Currently, many healthcare systems prioritize quantity of patient visits over the quality of those visits. However, it is clear that reducing the number of patients seen in a day, such as from 30 to 20 within an 8-hour shift, allows for more meaningful interactions, including valuable education for patients. The ongoing shortage of HCPs exacerbates this issue, forcing providers to see more patients regularly. Addressing this shortage requires proactive, multifaceted solutions, while also acknowledging the pervasive issue of provider burnout. To ensure quality patient education, healthcare systems may need to shift their focus toward a culture that values an adequate number of providers and prioritizes quality over quantity.

Insufficient Specialized Knowledge

HCPs may lack the specialized knowledge required for effective patient education, leading to potential issues such as duplication, omissions, or instruction from professionals who are not well-versed in the specific content area.[9] For instance, when explaining the impact of exercise on diabetes management, there is a risk of providing contradictory or inaccurate information.[10] Therefore, it is recommended that providers either acquire the necessary specialized knowledge or refer patients to another HCP who possesses expertise in the relevant field. In the management of patients with type II diabetes mellitus, PCPs may opt to refer patients to a diabetes educator specializing in diet plans. While PCPs are knowledgeable about the subject, this approach not only saves time for them but also ensures that patients receive high-quality education from a specialized educator.

Limited team-based approach

Effective patient care necessitates a profound understanding and consistent collaboration among HCPs managing shared patients. Unfortunately, patient education is often conducted in isolation, with healthcare professionals working independently and lacking TBA. This lacking may stem from a limited awareness of the educational content covered by other professions, resulting in a reluctance to delegate various educational topics.[11] Furthermore, this absence of TBA can negatively impact patient outcomes. For instance, in the case of managing a patient suspected of having sleep apnea, a PCP might refer the patient to a sleep laboratory for a sleep study. The challenge arises when, upon a sleep apnea diagnosis, some sleep laboratories provide continuous positive airway presssure (CPAP) machines and supplies while others do not. Without TBA, a patient may experience delays in obtaining a CPAP machine. Ideally, the PCP would refer the patient to the sleep laboratory, and upon the diagnosis of sleep apnea, the HCPs at the sleep laboratory educate the patient about the diagnosis and also provide the necessary CPAP equipment and instructions on usage. Subsequently, this information should be seamlessly communicated to the PCP for optimal patient care.

Redundant Education by Different Providers

It is a common occurrence for PCPs and other HCPs to spend a significant amount of time educating patients on the same topics. There is a general understanding that PCPs are responsible for patients' healthcare maintenance, which includes vaccinations. Specialists often streamline their communication by directing patients to their PCPs, stating, "Please consult your PCP about vaccines." This approach is efficient and direct. On the contrary, when a PCP refers a patient to a gastroenterologist (GI) for a screening colonoscopy, it becomes redundant for the PCP to extensively explain the procedure if the GI covers the same information during the initial consultation. Establishing a mutual understanding of each provider's specific role and expectations through transparent and comprehensive communication can eliminate redundant education. One consideration is for patients to carry a document listing all pertinent information. For instance, if a PCP refers a patient for a colonoscopy, the PCP should check the referral item, and the education about the colonoscopy procedure should be marked by whoever provides the information, whether it is the PCP or the GI specialist. Ideally, a checklist incorporating these tasks can be included in patients' charts, and different providers can initial their specific responsibilities in the EMRs. However, it is worth noting that not all EMRs are integrated to facilitate this practice.

Inconsistent Education Practices

Ensuring consistent information delivery by HCPs is crucial for bolstering their credibility and, by extension, the entire healthcare system. When information is inconsistent, patients not only become confused but also may lose trust in the healthcare system. This uncertainty can overwhelm patients, hindering the delivery of quality care and education.[12] For example, a patient with stable human immunodeficiency virus (HIV) and an undetectable viral load receives a recommendation from their HIV specialist to get the COVID-19 vaccine. If the PCP is unsure about this recommendation, they have options either to communicate directly with the HIV specialist or to take the time to research and communicate the vaccine recommendation accurately. However, if the PCP expresses uncertainty about the new vaccine and hesitates, patients may become confused and may even refuse the vaccine. Such instances not only contribute to patient confusion but also raise questions about the credibility of HCPs. Therefore, it is vital that HCPs in various settings consistently offer reliable information to shared patients, or at the very least, admit when they are unsure. If time constraints prevent communication with other providers or conducting research, honesty is key. In such cases, HCPs can transparently direct the patient to communicate directly with the expert in the field for accurate guidance.

High Provider Turnover

A high provider turnover can have adverse effects on patient education. Patients often find it disheartening to recount their medical history to numerous providers. With frequent turnover, patients may become hesitant to share their full medical background, potentially withholding crucial information. Utilizing EMR can mitigate this issue by enabling new providers to access patient charts, ask follow-up questions, and deliver appropriate patient education based on existing information. Generally, patients prefer the continuity of care provided by seeing the same HCP over an extended period. A high turnover may contribute to inconsistent education by different providers, as previously mentioned. Provider satisfaction, coupled with long-term commitment to one health system and continuous care for the same patients, can enhance both patient satisfaction and education.

Dependence on Electronic Medical Record for Patient Education

Following the adoption of EMR, incorporating patient education into the discharge summary has become a standard requirement for patient visits. HCPs now include patient education in the visit summary, assuming patients will read it. However, the effectiveness of this approach is uncertain, as it remains unclear how many patients actually engage with the provided education. While this method does save providers time, as they no longer need to spend extensive time educating patients on specific topics, it may not be as effective, given that some patients do not read the educational contents included in the visit summary. If HCPs choose to rely on patient education in the visit summary, it becomes crucial to remind patients of its importance and encourage them to read it. Despite the convenience, challenges arise due to the accessibility of both reliable and unreliable patient education online. Patients who encounter inaccurate information online may become confused when presented with accurate information by HCPs. It is essential to educate patients about the existence of unreliable online information and emphasize the importance of verifying such information with qualified HCPs.

Challenges Linked with Patients

While it is uncommon, patients experiencing lack of time is a possibility. Due to the high patient volume in provider schedule, some patients may have endured a lengthy wait for their appointments, causing potential delays in other plans for the day. These rushed patients might be less inclined to engage with patient education, even if the provider does an effective job. The time constraints often limit their ability to absorb information thoroughly.

Challenges with patient education can also stem from varying levels of education and language barriers. It is crucial for providers to gauge the patient's educational background and communicate accordingly. In instances where language barriers exist, even with interpretation services available, difficulties may arise in effectively conveying patient education. Providers should consider involving family members or friends when necessary. To address potential challenges, providers may ask patients with language barriers to recap their understanding of the education provided, ensuring accurate comprehension. This step is essential for confirming that patients have grasped the information correctly.

ETHICAL AND CULTURAL/DIVERSITY CONSIDERATIONS

In every aspect of medicine, including patient education, ethical and cultural diversity considerations are paramount. A compassionate attitude during patient education is a requirement necessary for all clinicians regardless of discipline. Compassion is a fundamental aspect of healthcare delivery, a sentiment echoed by many patients, families, clinicians, and policymakers alike.[13] The first principle of the American Medical Education underlines the necessity of compassion in care delivery. According to the Code of Ethics, "A physician shall be dedicated to providing competent medical care, with compassion and respect for human dignity and rights".[14] This expectation extends to other HCPs such as physician assistants, nurse practitioners, nurses, or pharmacists who are likewise required to practice with compassion. Hence, all clinicians are expected to provide proper care, including patient education. In this context, when encountering patients with language barriers or from different cultures, the expectation remains the same—they deserve an equitable treatment and appropriate patient education, just like any other patients.

FUTURE DIRECTIONS AND OPPORTUNITIES

A TBA to patient education is crucial for the future of healthcare. While some outpatient clinics have EMR access at certain Emergency Departments (EDs), others do not. The significance of EMR access becomes evident when a PCP sends a patient to the ED for an emergency, and subsequent monitoring and follow-ups are required. It is essential for every PCP to have access to ED EMRs, aligning with the long-term goal set with the adoption of EMRs in the US. Although progress has been made, there are still considerable ways to integrate all systems seamlessly.

In the realm of immunization, the California Immunization Registry (CAIR) stands out as a secure, confidential system that aids providers in tracking patient immunization records.[15] This system has replaced the traditional method of parents carrying immunization cards, providing an efficient means to maintain up-to-date records accessible from any clinic in California. Similarly, having a centralized database or a similar approach within existing EMRs for various patient conditions, including patient education, is highly recommended. This approach streamlines care, particularly for conditions requiring a multidisciplinary approach.

TBA is vital in preventing care fragmentation and unnecessary repetition of health services. A model like that of an ED and inpatient services within the same hospital system, serves as an effective example. In this model, information and patient education are documented in the same EMR, ensuring seamless communication among HCPs. This model can be adapted for outpatient clinics, addressing the current challenges where EMRs are not integrated, hindering proper patient care and education.

Improved communication between outpatient clinics is essential. For instance, when a PCP refers a patient to a specialist, effective communication between the 2 clinics should be established. A designated person responsible for overseeing this process can enhance communication. Each responsible provider should mark their initials on patient education items, creating accountability and ensuring that everyone is aware of who is responsible for each aspect of patient education. This approach is pivotal for achieving optimal patient outcomes.

When prioritizing patient education, several critical areas warrant consideration.

- *Role Clarification*

Every individual involved in patient education should possess a clear understanding of their role and the roles of others within the system.

- *Communication Infrastructure*

A reliable communication infrastructure is essential for patient education. An ideal approach is to implement a system similar to CAIR, as mentioned earlier. The most practical method involves utilizing existing EMRs within systems and ensuring their integration. Information technology and integrated documentation systems as highlighted can be employed to coordinate patient treatment and education.[6,16,17]

- *Shared Space for Collaboration*

Collaboration among all HCPs is paramount. Large outpatient clinics, housing multiple specialists and other providers, should convene regularly to discuss their respective roles. Introductions and periodic meetings—preferably every 3 to 6 months or at least annually—facilitate integration of the healthcare team. The current literature emphasizes the importance of these interactions for building rapport, trustful working relationships, and ultimately enhancing patient education.[11] Additionally, a shared space within the EMR can be utilized for communication regarding patient care and education.

- *Team-based Trust*

Optimum patient care, including education, requires trust among clinicians. Effective communication and trust-building are crucial, especially when a PCP refers a patient to a specialist. The specialist should communicate the prognosis with the PCP, and vice versa. This interprofessional trust fosters comprehensive patient care and contributes to better patient outcomes.

- *Organizational Support*

No effective patient education can occur without organizational support. When healthcare organizations prioritize quality patient care and support their providers and staff accordingly, it streamlines the process of delivering the best care and leads to positive outcomes. The literature underscores the importance of organizational support, advocating for resources and training opportunities to enhance future healthcare practices and policies for intracranial pressure in patient education.[11]

A recent systematic review conducted by Ho and colleagues suggested several recommendations for enhancing patient education:[11]

- *Team-based Interactions*

Create more opportunities for team-based interactions in patient education. This includes allocating designated time and space for participation in interprofessional bedside rounds and team discussions to foster shared goals and vision within the team. The collaboration of multidisciplinary HCPs to develop shared patient education resources and documentation processes is essential. Additionally, telecommunication can be utilized as an emerging platform for remote team-based meetings.

- *Standardized Patient Education Resources*

The collaboration of multidisciplinary HCPs is crucial for developing standardized patient education resources and documentation processes, facilitating the formalization of patient education.

- *Team-based Education*

Implement team-based education programs that focus on delivering team-based patient education. This approach aims to cultivate an understanding of the interdependent roles of multidisciplinary HCPs in providing patient-centered care.

- *Leadership Role Education*

Healthcare team members should be educated for their leadership role as coordinators of interprofessional teams leading patient education. Effective collaboration and communication with nurses are emphasized to facilitate necessary cooperation for patient education.

- *Other Considerations*

In addition, a team-based quality improvement (QI) training program within a large health system has demonstrated significant improvements in clinical quality measures. This program, designed to prepare individuals from various departments and professions within the health system to lead QI, involved broad stakeholder input and rigorous evaluation. Other large health systems may adopt a similar approach to train HCPs across specialties, settings, and backgrounds to lead QI.[18] Furthermore, future QI projects and research are highly recommended concerning the TBA to patient education. Given the evolving nature of healthcare delivery, timely and insightful findings are vital for providing optimal care to patients.

SUMMARY

The current evidence unequivocally indicates that delivering effective patient education is crucial for achieving positive health outcomes. It is also widely acknowledged that healthcare is a collaborative endeavor, necessitating all healthcare professionals to unite, cooperate, and educate patients collectively for optimal results. Despite this awareness among HPCs about the benefits of thorough patient education, numerous challenges exist within the healthcare system when it comes to implementing a team-based approach to patient education. Various models for team-based patient education have been proposed and put into practice. However, no single model fits all scenarios, emphasizing the importance of customization based on different team dynamics. Utilizing new technologies and online platforms appears to be a promising avenue for delivering comprehensive patient education. Nevertheless, careful consideration is essential to address any potential gaps or shortcomings in this approach. Further research is warranted in this domain to refine and enhance patient education practices, ensuring they meet the evolving needs of patients and healthcare teams alike.

CLINICS CARE POINTS

- Collaborative Education: Primary care providers and specialists should work together to provide the best education to their patients.

- Specialized Expertise: Defer patient education to specialists/experts when the topic is beyond the primary care provider's scope.
- Utilize Resources: If time is limited, involve others in patient education. For instance, refer patients to a nutritional counselor if there's not enough time to educate them about healthy diet and nutrition.
- Encourage Communication: Urge patients to communicate with both primary care providers and specialists to ensure that everyone involved in their care is aligned on managing their medical conditions.
- Address Time Constraints: If providers struggle with time constraints for patient education, discuss the issue with organizational leadership.
- Promote Education Culture: Foster a culture within the organization that prioritizes patient education for improved patient outcomes.
- Role Model for Future Clinicians: When training or precepting the next generation of clinicians, demonstrate that patient education is an essential part of comprehensive patient care.

DISCLOSURE

The authors have nothing to disclose.

REFERENCES

1. Rawlinson C, Carron T, Cohidon C, et al. An overview of reviews on interprofessional collaboration in primary care: barriers and facilitators. Int J Integrated Care 2021. https://doi.org/10.5334/ijic.5589.
2. Geese F, Schmitt K-U. Interprofessional collaboration in complex patient care transition: a qualitative multi-perspective analysis. Healthcare 2023;11(3):359. Available at: https://www.mdpi.com/2227-9032/11/3/359 https://mdpi-res.com/d_attachment/healthcare/healthcare-11-00359/article_deploy/ healthcare-11-00359-v2.pdf?version=1675742929.
3. Bosch B, Mansell H. Interprofessional collaboration in health care: Lessons to be learned from competitive sports. Can Pharm J 2015;148(4):176–9 (In eng).
4. Hopkins K, Sinsky CA. Taking team-based care to the next level. Fam Pract Manag 2022;29(3):25–31 (In eng), Available at: https://www.aafp.org/pubs/fpm/issues/2022/0500/p25.pdf.
5. Braam A, Buljac-Samardzic M, Hilders C, et al. Collaboration between physicians from different medical specialties in hospital settings: a systematic review. J Multidiscip Healthc 2022;15:2277–300 (In eng).
6. Vos JFJ, Boonstra A, Kooistra A, et al. The influence of electronic health record use on collaboration among medical specialties. BMC Health Serv Res 2020;20(1):676 (In eng).
7. D'Amour D, Ferrada-Videla M, San Martin Rodriguez L, et al. The conceptual basis for interprofessional collaboration: core concepts and theoretical frameworks. J Interprof Care 2005;19(Suppl 1):116–31.
8. Wei H, Horns P, Sears SF, et al. A systematic meta-review of systematic reviews about interprofessional collaboration: facilitators, barriers, and outcomes. J Interprof Care 2022;36(5):735–49.
9. Causey-Upton R, Howell DM, Kitzman PH, et al. Orthopaedic nurses' perceptions of preoperative education for total knee replacement. Orthop Nurs 2020;39(4):227–37 (In eng).

10. Litchfield I, Andrews RC, Narendran P, et al. Patient and healthcare professionals perspectives on the delivery of exercise education for patients with type 1 diabetes. Front Endocrinol (Lausanne) 2019;10:76 (In eng).
11. Ho JT, See MTA, Tan AJQ, et al. Healthcare professionals' experiences of interprofessional collaboration in patient education: a systematic review. Patient Educ Couns 2023;116:107965 (In eng).
12. Papadakos J, Giannopoulos E, Forbes L, et al. Reinventing the wheel: The incidence and cost implication of duplication of effort in patient education materials development. Patient Educ Couns 2021;104(6):1398–405 (In eng).
13. Malenfant S, Jaggi P, Hayden KA, et al. Compassion in healthcare: an updated scoping review of the literature. BMC Palliat Care 2022;21(1):80 (In eng).
14. Riddick FA Jr. The code of medical ethics of the american medical association. Ochsner J 2003;5(2):6–10 (In eng).
15. Health CDoP. California immunization registry. California Department of Public Health. Available at: https://www.cdph.ca.gov/Programs/CID/DCDC/CAIR/Pages/CAIR-updates-about.aspx.
16. Johnson AM, Brimhall AS, Johnson ET, et al. A systematic review of the effectiveness of patient education through patient portals. JAMIA Open 2023;6(1). https://doi.org/10.1093/jamiaopen/ooac085.
17. Honavar SG. Electronic medical records - The good, the bad and the ugly. Indian J Ophthalmol 2020;68(3):417–8 (In eng).
18. O'Leary KJ, Knoten CA, Fant AL, et al. Implementation and effects of a team-based quality improvement training program across a health system: the northwestern medicine academy for quality and safety improvement. Jt Comm J Qual Patient Saf 2021;47(8):481–8 (In eng).

Promoting Health Equity and Social Justice

Donna F. Murray, DMSc, MS, PA-C[a],*, Richard D. Ball, DHSc, MPH, PA-C[b]

KEYWORDS

- Social justice • Health equity • Health disparities • Social determinants of health

KEY POINTS

- This article helps us in defining health, health care disparities, and health equity.
- It explains what is meant by social determinants of health, structural racism, discrimination, and their impact on the health care system.
- This article also discusses the goals of Healthy People 2030.
- It also discusses social justice, cultural sensitivity, and cultural competency in health care delivery.
- It also discusses strategies used to promote Health Equity and Social Justice.

INTRODUCTION

The emergence of the COVID-19 pandemic served as a catalyst for our nation, revealing the intricate links among socioeconomics, race, and health outcomes. As a nation, we were forced to reckon with the reality that health disparities persist and there is a direct correlation between access to care and the roles classism, racism, and heath literacy play in health outcomes. Many of our patients faced the realities created by the pandemic as they were forced to navigate the complexities associated with limited health literacy, and access to care as well as socioeconomics. During this public health crisis, there was little time to provide education to patients. However, we have a responsibility now to educate patients and provide them with the tools they need to self-advocate.

In the United States and in many countries around the world, the impetus for health care and public health initiatives stems from a need to address issues of disparities that pose a threat to the country and the government's stability and viability. Governments have long recognized that a reasonably healthy population is important to their goals and objectives for governing.[1] As patients develop a clear understanding of community engagement as a driver of the social justice movement, they will realize the need for collaborative strategies to combat the inequities that exist. In short, as

[a] Morehouse School of Medicine PA Studies Program, 720 Westview Drive Southwest, Atlanta, GA 30310, USA; [b] Florida International University MPAS Program, 11200 Southwest 8th Street, MARC Suite 238, Miami, FL 33199, USA
* Corresponding author.
E-mail address: dfmpac0896@gmail.com

Physician Assist Clin 9 (2024) 515–526
https://doi.org/10.1016/j.cpha.2024.06.002 **physicianassistant.theclinics.com**
2405-7991/24/© 2024 Elsevier Inc. All rights are reserved, including those for text and data mining, AI training, and similar technologies.

we examine the intersectionality of health equity and social justice, we must consider the role of government in setting policy and the role of social activism in addressing health disparities and creating an environment in which health for all is realized.

SOCIAL JUSTICE

Social justice is defined as the fair treatment and equitable status of all individuals and social groups within a society. The term is also used to refer to social political, and economic institutions, laws, or policies that collectively afford such fairness and equity. The term commonly applied to movements that seed equity, inclusion, self-determination for historically oppressed, exploited, or marginalized populations. In theoretic terms, social justice is often understood to be equivalent to justice itself.[2]

HEALTH, HEALTH EQUITY, AND HEALTH DISPARITIES

The World Health Organization (WHO) defines health as a state of complete physical mental and social well-being and not merely the absence of disease or infirmity. Additionally, the preamble to the Constitution of WHO outlines a set of 8 principles that include enjoyment of the highest standard of health is one of the fundamental rights of every human being without distinction of race, religion, political belief, economic, or social condition.[1]

Health equity is the state in which everyone has a fair and just opportunity to attain their highest level of health.[3] The Healthy People 2030 Initiative defines health equity as the "attainment of the highest levels of health for all people. Achieving health equity requires valuing everyone equally with the focus on ongoing society efforts to address avoidable inequalities, historical and contemporary injustices, and the elimination of health and health care disparities."[4]

According to the Britannica Dictionary, disparity is defined as a noticeable and often unfair difference between people or things.[5] A health care disparity is a difference between population groups in the way they access, experience, and receive health care.[6] Health disparities are preventable differences in the burden of disease, injury, violence, or opportunities to achieve optimal health that are experienced by populations that have been disadvantaged by their social or economic status, geographic location, and environment.[7]

These disparities are often rooted in social determinants such as income, education, race, ethnicity, gender, and geographic location.

The issue of health disparities and their determinants has been a subject of study and concern for many years, and as a result, the existence of disparities in health and health care delivery has become well established in the field of public health and health care policy. In the United States, the discussion of health disparities has been a prominent feature in health care reform and efforts to improve the equity of health care access and outcomes. Various reports, studies, and organizations have contributed to our understanding of health disparities and have played a role in shaping how we define and address them.[8,9]

Health care delivery is not experienced equitably by all populations. In many instances, our health care system distributes services inefficiently and unevenly across populations. This inequity and inefficiency result in some Americans not receiving the care they need, receiving care that causes harm, receiving care that is delivered too late, and receiving care that is provided without full consideration of a patient's preferences and values.[8,9]

Various government agencies, research institutions, and advocacy organizations have contributed to raising awareness about these disparities and seeking solutions to address them. Disparities can be observed across a wide range of health indicators, that is, life expectancy, infant mortality, chronic disease prevalence, and health care utilization patterns. These disparities may occur for a variety of reasons, including differences in access to care, social determinants, provider biases, poor provider–patient communication, and poor health literacy.[8,9]

SOCIAL DETERMINANTS OF HEALTH

In 1979, Surgeon General Julius Richmond issued a landmark report titled *"Healthy People: The Surgeon General's Report on Health Promotion and Disease Prevention."* In 1980, the Office of Disease Prevention and Health Promotion implemented the Healthy People 1990 Initiative. The Healthy People Initiative is a program that sets measurable objectives to improve the health and well-being of people nationwide. It was first launched in 1980 and has since been updated every decade to address the latest public health priorities and challenges.[5,10]

Healthy People 2000, 2010, and 2020 included achieving health equity and the elimination of health disparities among the overarching goals of the initiative.[11] Healthy People 2030, launched in August 2020, is the fifth and current iteration of the Healthy People initiative. It builds on knowledge gained over the last 4 decades and has an increased focus on health equity, social determinants of health, and health literacy with a new focus on well-being.[10,12] Social determinants of health as determined by Healthy People 2030 are the conditions in the environments where people are born, live, learn, work, play, worship, and age that affect a wide range of health, functioning, and quality-of-life outcomes and risks.[8,9] Additionally, providers must recognize the relationship among class, education, occupation, and income as they engage patients and that class may impact the patient's ability to navigate society as a whole.[13] At each patient encounter, health care providers should take the opportunity to discuss social determinants of health as they impact the patient's daily life or the lives of family members. This will provide an opportunity for patients to articulate matters that are impacting their well-being.

Five Domains of Social Determinants of Health and How to Approach Each One during a Patient Encounter:

1. Economic stability/poverty—Do you have difficulty with housing, food, paying for utilities, and paying for medication?
2. Education access and quality—What level of education have you achieved? What are your thoughts about advancing your education? Do you have access to a local library?
3. Health care access and quality—How far do you have to travel to medical appointments? Do you have access to transportation?
4. Neighborhood and built environment—Do you live in a community where you feel safe walking alone? Are you aware of gun violence in your community?
5. Social and community context—Do you live in a community where there are friends, family, church, synagogue, temple, and recreation activities?

Health care providers should also engage patient regarding the social determinants of mental health. They are also grouped into 5 domains each influenced by marginalization, discrimination, segregation, poverty, poor education, inequality, violence, isolation, and loneliness. The 5 domains include racism, ethnicity, age, gender, and access to services.[14,15] Additional variables that contribute to the health disparities, mental health disparities, and social determinants of health that overlap with the 5 domains delineated earlier include[8,9,14,16,17]

• Homophobia/LGBTQ+ Bias	• Access to nutritious foods
• Language differences	• Polluted air and water
• Housing status	• Transportation
• Lack of sick leave	• Domestic violence
• Childcare needs	• Substance abuse
• Unemployment	• Immigration status
• Lack of insurance or inadequate coverage	• Physical disability

Environmental health risks such as the degradation of the overall living environment including air, water, and soil pollution are more prevalent in low-income, racial, and ethnic minority communities. Research also demonstrates that needed health services such as hospitals, clinics, private, and group practices have a very limited presence in areas that have populations with predominance of poor and minoritized groups. Insufficient transportation is another factor that impacts access to health care for members of these groups living in these marginalized areas. People in hazardous low-paying occupations are disproportionately exposed to physical hazards, crime, violence, and minoritized individuals.[18]

Discriminatory laws, polices, and practices have also been noted to be factors in disparate health care. The foundations for the disparities seen in Americans of African descent date back to chattel slavery, the implementation of "Jim Crow" laws in the immediate post-slavery era, particularly in southern states. These laws and policies were implemented nationwide on the heels of significant Supreme Court decisions in support of these laws. As a result, discrimination and disparities proliferated in the form of[19–21]:

• Housing (Redlining, Sun-down Towns)	• Access to health care
• Black codes	• Environmental racism
• Racial covenants	• Bank loans of housing and businesses
• Racial property seizures	• Homestead Act Exclusion
• White domestic terrorism/racial massacres	• New deal exclusions
• Police brutality	• Federal Housing Administration (FHA) mortgage exclusion
• War on drugs	• Government Issue (G.I.) Bill Exclusions
• Denial of voting rights	• Medical experimentation
• Mass incarceration	

CONSEQUENCES OF HEALTH CARE DISPARITIES AND PROMISES OF IMPROVED HEALTH LITERACY

Health care disparities can have far-reaching and significant consequences for individuals, communities, and society. Addressing health care disparities is not only a matter of improving individual health outcomes but is also crucial for building a more just, equitable, and resilient society. Efforts to eliminate disparities must involve comprehensive, systemic approaches that address health care-specific factors, patient health education and health literacy, as well as the broader social determinants of health.

Some of the key consequences include[21]

• Poor health outcomes	• Health care access barriers
• Reduced quality of care	• Healthcare deserts
• Health inequities	• Mental health consequences
• Economic burden	• Social injustice and inequality
• Lost productivity	• Reduced trust in health care system
• Health care system strain	• Moral and ethical concerns
• Social and economic disadvantage	

STRATEGIES TO ADDRESS HEALTH CARE DISPARITIES THROUGH PATIENT EDUCATION

As citizens and community members, we can join the effort to ensure that all people have equitable access to resources to maintain and manage their physical and mental health. Community-based and faith-based organizations, employers, health care systems and providers, public health agencies, policymakers, and others play a key part in promoting fair access to health, improving opportunity, and ensuring that all communities can thrive.[21]

Health care providers can play a pivotal role in improving health literacy and empowering patients to play an active role in combatting health care disparities in the local communities. Patients can organize members of their communities and implement initiatives that focus on improving access to health care, increasing health literacy, and addressing social determinants of health.

1. Define social justice and health care disparities:
   - Explain what social justice means in the context of health care, emphasizing the fair and equitable distribution of resources, opportunities, and health care services.
2. Provide statistics and examples:
   - Share relevant statistics and real-life examples of health care disparities to illustrate the extent of the issue. Highlight disparities based on race, ethnicity, socioeconomic status, gender, and other factors.
3. Discuss root causes:
   - Explore the root causes of health care disparities, including systemic issues such as discrimination, unequal access to education and economic opportunities, and implicit biases within the health care system.
4. Highlight the impact on health outcomes:
   - Emphasize how health care disparities can lead to differences in health outcomes and quality of care for individuals from marginalized communities.
5. Promote cultural competence:
   - Encourage health care providers to be culturally competent by understanding and respecting the cultural backgrounds, beliefs, and values of their patients. This can improve communication and trust.
6. Advocate for health literacy:
   - Stress the importance of health literacy and its role in empowering individuals to make informed decisions about their health care. Provide resources and tools to enhance health literacy.
7. Encourage patient advocacy:
   - Teach patients how to advocate for themselves within the health care system. This includes knowing their rights, asking questions, seeking second opinions, and reporting any discriminatory practices.
8. Address implicit bias:
   - Discuss the concept of implicit bias within health care and encourage patients to speak up if they feel they are being treated unfairly. Promote open communication with health care providers.
9. Promote community engagement:
   - Encourage patients to get involved in community organizations and initiatives that address health care disparities. Collective action can bring about positive change.
10. Share resources:
    - Provide patients with resources, such as Web sites, articles, and organizations dedicated to addressing health care disparities and promoting social justice in health care.

11. Utilize multimedia and storytelling:
   - Use multimedia, such as videos and personal stories, to engage patients emotionally and help them connect with the realities of health care disparities.
12. Encourage a holistic approach to health:
   - Emphasize the importance of addressing social determinants of health, such as education, housing, and employment, in addition to medical care.

By educating patients about social justice and health care disparities, we empower them to actively participate in their health care and advocate for a more equitable and just health care system.

Strategies that local communities can consider include the following:[4]

1. Promote community health education.
2. Promote community health fairs and screenings.
3. Establish new social support services and support and expand existing social support programs.
4. Partner with community-based and faith-based organizations.
5. Implement and support youth outreach and education.
6. Explore and promote telehealth services to increase access to health care.
7. Advocate for local policies that address health care disparities.
8. Collect and analyze local health data to identify specific disparities and target interventions effectively.

Health systems in partnership with employers can play a significant role in addressing health care disparities by implementing policies and initiatives that prioritize employee health and well-being. By implementing these strategies, employers can contribute to creating a workplace culture that values and prioritizes the health of all employees, helping to mitigate health care disparities and promote overall well-being.

Strategies employers can adopt to help reduce health care disparities include the following:[21]

1. Provide comprehensive and affordable health insurance coverage.
2. Implement workplace wellness programs that focus on promoting healthy lifestyles.
3. Provide cultural competency training for health care providers and staff.
4. Provide confidential culturally sensitive and accessible counseling and support services to address mental health issues, stress, and work–life balance.
5. Implement flexible work schedules or telecommuting options to accommodate employees' health care needs and appointments without fear of negative consequences.
6. Promote health literacy by providing educational materials, workshops, and resources.
7. Establish employee resource groups focused on health and wellness to provide a platform for employees to share information, experiences, and resources.
8. Foster a workplace culture that promotes diversity, equity, inclusion, and belonging.
9. Collaborate with local health care providers, clinics, and community organizations to extend health care resources to employees and their families.
10. Conduct regular health assessments to identify prevalent health concerns within the workforce and tailor interventions accordingly.

Health systems can also partner with communities to address health care disparities by implementing strategies that ensure equitable access to high-quality care for all patients.

Actions health care delivery systems can take include the following:[21]

1. Provide ongoing cultural competency training for health care professionals.
2. Provide interpreters and translated materials.
3. Engage with local communities to understand their unique health care needs and preferences.
4. Allocate resources strategically to address disparities, with a focus on underserved and poor communities.
5. Implement patient navigation programs to assist individuals in scheduling appointments and accessing necessary services.

Public health agencies play a crucial role in addressing health care disparities by implementing policies, programs, and initiatives that target the root causes of disparities. By taking these actions, public health agencies can contribute significantly to reducing health care disparities and advancing health equity in communities.

Actions public health agencies can take include the following:[21,22]

1. Collect, analyze, and report health data to identify and monitor health care disparities and tailor interventions accordingly.
2. Develop and implement health equity initiatives that explicitly aim to eliminate disparities.
3. Foster partnerships with community organizations, advocacy groups, and local stakeholders to address specific health concerns.
4. Design culturally competent and linguistically appropriate interventions and educational materials.
5. Advocate for policies that address systemic inequalities and the social determinants of health.
6. Promote and facilitate access to preventive services, including vaccinations, screenings, and early detection programs.
7. Implement health literacy programs to improve understanding of health information among diverse populations.
8. Promote diversity within the public health workforce to increase representation and enhance cultural competence.
9. Advocate for policies at all levels of government that advance health equity and address structural determinants of disparities.

State, tribal, local, and territorial governments play a critical role in addressing health care disparities. By implementing these strategies, each group can contribute to reducing health care disparities and fostering health equity within their jurisdictions.

Strategies they can initiate include the following:[21]

1. Mandate the collection and reporting of health data to identify and monitor health care disparities.
2. Develop and implement standards for culturally competent health care services.
3. Engage with local communities and tribal nations to understand their unique health care needs.
4. Promote diversity within the health care workforce.
5. Develop and implement policies that explicitly address health disparities and promote health equity.
6. Invest in underserved communities.
7. Expand the use of community health workers who can bridge cultural and linguistic gaps.

8. Establish and strengthen partnerships with tribal nations to address the unique health care needs of indigenous populations.

PROMOTING SOCIAL JUSTICE TO FOSTER HEALTH EQUITY

Social justice in principle is concerned with equal treatment, equal access, equal rights, and equal opportunities for all regardless of race, ethnicity, gender, class, or socioeconomic status. As a society, it is the responsibility of everyone to ensure this treatment within the health care delivery system. However, there are inequities in health care that exist and are experienced by patients who are the direct result of unequal access to resources in underserved and marginalized communities. Creating awareness for patients that the inequities that exist are rooted in policies, and structure that is directly tied to the social determinants of health is critical to empowering them to become agents of change. To address these inequities, the conditions that lead to them must be addressed. By educating our patients, they can work to change the conditions that impact their care and care of others in their communities.

Structural Racism

In October 2020, the American Public Health Association (APHA) released a statement addressing structural racism identifying it as a public health crisis. Racism is defined as a pervasive system of power based on the social construct of race, that is, ideological notions of the inherent superiority of non-Hispanic "Whites" and inherent inferiority of people of color that operated across multiple levels to unjustly advantage Whites and unjustly disadvantage person of color.[23] The fight against structural racism begins with examining one's own beliefs and biases. Recognizing internal beliefs is the beginning of elimination of the power structure that is the root cause of disparate care experienced by people of color.

Access to Care and Health Care Systems

Systemic change leads to improved access to care. Access to care is related to level of education and health literacy, where individuals live, including environmental factors, and where individuals work. The health of individuals is impacted by where individuals live and their access to exercise-friendly and safer, nonviolent communities. Health care systems changes that would substantially impact access are universal health coverage and the elimination of bias in the delivery of diagnostic and therapeutic interventions.[24] Community engagement and support of local health care organizations that provide care to underserved communities can contribute to eliminating the barriers to care and promoting improved health literacy in those communities.

Criminal Justice and Violence in Marginalized Communities

Research suggests that well-being suffers when one is negatively exposed to the legal system.[25] Members of marginalized communities are disproportionately affected by over-policing, mass incarceration, and violence. For decades, the criminal justice system has been involved in perpetuating racism and the structure has created racialized health disparities.[26] Giving voice to the "voiceless" where there is weaponization of the legal system can be impactful. Encouraging patients to support politicians, political activists, and social justice champions committed to dismantling the system can have a significant impact. Creating and awareness of businesses and corporations that invest in the for-profit prison industrial complex can have a financial impact on the contributions these companies have on mass incarceration.

Voting Rights

Communities of color are increasingly impacted by poor health outcomes. Those that are impacted disproportionately by changes in districts are also disproportionately impacted by health disparities. There is a direct correlation among decreased access to voting, structural inequities, and a decreased interest in those suffering from chronic disease. In 2022, the American Medical Association passed a policy resolution declaring voting a social determinant of health.[26] Political activism that stems from patient education and increased health literacy can be a driver of the social justice movement. Voter registration efforts led by health systems along can empower those in marginalized communities while helping to build political power for communities that traditionally do not participate in the political process.

CULTURAL SENSITIVITY AND CULTURAL COMPETENCY IN HEALTH CARE

Culture has been defined as an integrated pattern of human behavior that includes the thoughts, communications, actions, customs, beliefs, values, and institutions of a racial, ethnic, religious, or social group. Cultural competency in health care describes the ability of health care workers and health care systems to provide care to patients with diverse values, beliefs, and behaviors, including the tailoring of health care delivery to meet patients' social, cultural, and linguistic needs.[27–29] Cultural competency also takes into consideration the cultural belief systems of the cause of disease and illness and their relationship of health and healing and attitudes toward seeking help from health care providers.[30]

People generally tend to assume that a common culture is shared between members of racial, linguistic, and religious groups. Large groups of people in this country may share common historical and geographic experiences; however, individuals within these groups may share nothing beyond physical appearance, language, or spiritual beliefs.[27–29]

Medicine has evolved into a culture with its own set of rules, customs, beliefs, and practices that promote scientific rationality with an emphasis on objectivity that can, at times, conflict with patients' beliefs and practices. Providers, like most people, tend to understand culture in its broadest sense and usually interpret it as something that groups possess. A provider's cultural background is likely to influence his/her practice of medicine just as much as a patient's cultural background will influence his/her behavior in interactions with the health care system.[28,29]

An integral part of providing culturally competent care is understanding how factors such as geography, environment, religion, gender, socioeconomic status, and education affect how a person seeks and uses medical care, as well as his/her group's historical relationship with the health care system. The need for cultural sensitivity and cultural competency education for health care providers is evidenced by the persistence of health care disparities that impact ethnic and racial minorities in this country.[27–29]

SUMMARY

Health care disparities in the United States represent a complex and deeply rooted issue that requires sustained attention and comprehensive solutions. Achieving health equity demands a multifaceted approach that includes dismantling discriminatory practices, improving access to quality health care in underserved areas, and addressing social determinants of health. Emphasizing cultural competence, increasing diversity in the health care workforce, and promoting health literacy are integral components of reducing disparities. Ultimately, achieving health care equity is not only a moral imperative, but it is also essential for the overall well-being of the nation.

This study highlights the intricate relationship among social justice, health equity, health care disparities, and their collective impact on patient education. We must consider the patient at the center as we address health equity and health disparities. Empowering patients with health education and health literacy while encouraging them to become instruments of the social justice movement will facilitate change to improve systems of care. Achieving meaningful progress in reducing health care disparities requires a comprehensive approach that addresses social determinants, recognizes intersectionality, and incorporates the principles of social justice into policy and practice. By doing so, our society can move closer to realizing a health care system that upholds the values of fairness, equity, and inclusivity for all.

CLINICS CARE POINTS

- Increased health literacy improves the patient's ability to self-advocate in the face of health disparities.
- Patients must actively participate in the social justice movement to help create health equity and eliminate health disparities.
- Systemic change can happen when there is a comprehensive approcach that addresses social determinants of health and change in policy.

DISCLOSURE

The authors have nothing to disclose.

REFERENCES

1. Constitution of the world health organization 49th edition. 2020. Available at: https://www.who.int/about/governance/constitution. [Accessed 23 October 2023].
2. https://www.britannica.com/topics/social-justice.
3. Center for the Study of Social Policy. Key equity terms and concepts: A glossary for shared understanding. Available at: https://cssp.org/resource/key-equity-terms-and-concepts-a-glossary-for-shared-understanding. [Accessed 22 September 2023].
4. https://health.gov/healthypeople/priority-areas/health-equity-healthy-people-2030. [Accessed 31 December 2023].
5. The Britannica Dictionary. Definition of disparity. Available at: https://www.britannica.com/dictionary/disparity. [Accessed 19 October 2023].
6. Definition of Healthcare Disparity. National Healthcare Quality and Disparities Report. Available at: https://www.ncbi.nlm.nih.gov/books/NBK578532/. [Accessed 13 September 2023].
7. Braveman P, Arkin E, Orleans T, et al. What is Health Equity?. 2018. Available at: https://behavioralpolicy.org/wp-content/uploads/2018/12/What-is-Health-Equity.pdf. [Accessed 19 October 2023].
8. Healthy People 2030. Social Determinants of Health. Available at: https://health.gov/healthypeople/priority-areas/social-determinants-health. [Accessed 27 October 2023].

9. Healthy People 2030: Reduce bullying of lesbian, gay, or bisexual high school students — LGBT. Available at: https://health.gov/healthypeople/objectives-and-data/browse-objectives/lgbt/reduce-bullying-lesbian-gay-or-bisexual-high-school-students-lgbt-05. [Accessed 11 October 2023].

10. Healthy People 2030. Objectives. Available at: https://health.gov/healthypeople/objectives-and-data/browse-objectives. [Accessed 17 November 2023].

11. Healthy People 2020. Overview of Health Disparities. Available at: https://www.cdc.gov/nchs/healthy_people/hp2020/health-disparities.htm. [Accessed 23 August 2023].

12. Healthy People 2030 National Health Initiatives. Available at: https://health.gov/our-work/national-health-initiatives/healthy-people/healthy-people-2030. [Accessed 23 September 2023].

13. Čirjak A. Does the United States have a Class System? Society 2020. Available at: https://www.worldatlas.com/articles/does-the-united-states-have-a-class-system.html. [Accessed 20 September 2023].

14. Social determinants of mental health in children and youth American psychological association manual. Available at: https://www.psychiatry.org/getattachment/a03e07c5-bba9-4ac7-b434-9183b1e0b730/Resource-Document-Social-Determinants-of-Mental-Health. [Accessed 30 September 2023].

15. Chapman EN, Kaatz A, Carnes M. Physicians and implicit bias: how doctors may unwittingly perpetuate health care disparities. JGIM 2013;128:1504. Available at: https://www.ncbi.nlm.nih.gov/pmc/articles/PMC3797360/. [Accessed 30 September 2023].

16. Krahn GL, Walker DK, Correa-De-Araujo R. Persons with disabilities as an unrecognized health disparity population. Am J Public Health 2015;105(Suppl 2):S198–206.

17. American Psychological Association. Discrimination: What it is, and how to cope. 2019. Available at: https://www.apa.org/topics/racism-bias-discrimination/types-stress. [Accessed 13 November 2023].

18. Impact of Racism on our Nation's Health. 2021. Available at: https://www.cdc.gov/minorityhealth/racism-disparities/impact-of-racism.html. [Accessed 23 October 2023].

19. Brian DS, Stith AY, Nelson AR. Unequal Treatment: Confronting Racial and Ethnic Disparities in Health Care. Institute of medicine committee on understanding and eliminating racial and ethnic disparities in health care. 2003. Available at: https://pubmed.ncbi.nlm.nih.gov/250323861. [Accessed 13 October 2023].

20. Paradies Y. A systematic review of empirical research on self-reported racism and health. Int J Epidemiol 2006;35(4):888–901. Available at: https://academic.oup.com/ije/article/35/4/888/686369. [Accessed 12 November 2023].

21. Jack L Jr. Advancing Health Equity, Eliminating Health Disparities, and Improving Population Health. Prev Chronic Dis 2021;18:210264. Available at: https://www.cdc.gov/pcd/issues/2021/21_0264.htm. [Accessed 1 December 2023].

22. The future of public health, summary of the public health system in the United States institute of medicine committee for the study of the future of public health. Washington DC: National Academies Press; 1988. Available at: https://www.ncbi.nlm.nih.gov/books/NBK218212/https://www.ncbi.nlm.nih.gov/books/NBK218212/. [Accessed 12 October 2023].

23. Available at: https://www.apha.org/policies-and-advocacy/public-health-policy-statements/policy-database/2021/01/13/structural-racism-is-a-public-health-crisis. [Accessed 3 January 2024].

24. Satcher D, Fryer GE, McCann J, et al. What If We Were Equal? A Comparison of the Black-White Mortality Gap in 1960 and 2000. 2000. Available at: https://www.researchgate.net/profile/George-Rust/publication/7976375. [Accessed 29 September 2023].

25. Available at: https://blog.petrieflom.law.harvard.edu/2021/09/10/health-justice-criminal-legal-system/. [Accessed 3 January 2024].

26. Available at: https://catalyst.nejm.org/doi/full/10.1056/CAT.22.0368. [Accessed 3 January 2024].

27. Handtke BS, Mösko M. Culturally competent healthcare: A scoping review of strategies implemented in healthcare organizations and a model of culturally competent healthcare provision. 2019. Available at: https://doi.org/10.1371/journal.pone.0219971. [Accessed 27 August 2023].

28. Sara Heath. What Does Cultural Competence Mean for Healthcare Providers? 2020. Available at: https://patientengagementhit.com/news/what-does-cultural-competence-mean-for-healthcare-providers. [Accessed 17 September 2023].

29. Monica E, Peek MD, MPH MS. Increasing Representation of Black Primary Care Physicians—A Critical Strategy to Advance Racial. Health Equity JAMA 2023; 6(4):e236678. Available at: https://jamanetwork.com/journals/jamanetworkopen/fullarticle/2803903. [Accessed 27 August 2023].

30. Office of Management and Budget. Revisions to the Standards for the Classification of Federal Data on Race and Ethnicity. 2001. Available at: https://orwh.od.nih.gov/toolkit/other-relevant-federal-policies/OMB-standards. [Accessed 13 September 2023].

Patient Education in Chronic Disease Management

Edward Adinkrah, MD, MPH, PMP*

KEYWORDS

- Chronic diseases • Patient education • Lifestyle modifications
- Medication adherence • Self-management • Digital tools

KEY POINTS

- For successful management of chronic diseases, it is important to prioritize patient education that highlights the significance of adhering to prescribed medications, making lifestyle changes, and enhancing self-management capabilities.
- Evidence-based approaches and digital health interventions play a critical role in enhancing patient education and disease management outcomes.
- Challenges, such as health literacy, resource accessibility, and cultural sensitivity, need to be addressed to optimize patient education efforts.
- Future directions include leveraging innovations in digital health and personalized medicine to further enhance chronic disease management.
- Health care providers are encouraged to integrate patient-focused educational strategies into treatment plans, using technology and proven techniques to assist patients in managing their long-term health concerns.

INTRODUCTION
Navigating the Complexities of Chronic Diseases

This article explores the complexities of managing chronic diseases. Chronic health conditions, such as diabetes, heart diseases, and persistent respiratory conditions, pose significant challenges for health care systems worldwide.[1–3] These ailments are among the causes of death and illness globally, affecting millions of people and placing burdens on individuals, families, and communities.[4,5] The management of such diseases demands a multifaceted approach that goes beyond medical treatments to encompass patient education, lifestyle modifications, and continuous support.[6] The intricate nature of managing chronic illnesses highlights the need for strategies that empower patients to actively engage in their own well-being.

Charles R. Drew University of Medicine and Science, 1731 East 120th Street, Los Angeles, CA 90059, USA
* 38713 Tierra Subida Avenue #200-628, Palmdale, CA 93551.
E-mail address: edwardadinkrah1@cdrewu.edu

Physician Assist Clin 9 (2024) 527–540
https://doi.org/10.1016/j.cpha.2024.05.005
physicianassistant.theclinics.com
2405-7991/24/© 2024 Elsevier Inc. All rights are reserved, including those for text and data mining, AI training, and similar technologies.

The Evolution and Impact of Patient Education

The evolution of patient education from a paternalistic model to a cornerstone of modern health care reflects significant shifts in health and wellness perspectives.[7] Initially rooted in nineteenth-century public health movements, patient education aimed to spread knowledge on hygiene and disease prevention.[8] The twentieth century saw a paradigm shift toward recognizing the importance of patient autonomy and the emergence of patient-centered care, fundamentally changing the approach to patient education.[9]

In the digital age, although patient education faces challenges in information reliability and validity, it remains imperative for enhancing patient and community knowledge, skills, engagement in self-care, and overall improvement in patients' health care experience.[10]

Embracing Self-Management and Lifestyle Modifications

Self-management or care is focused on equipping patients with knowledge and skills required to make informed daily health decisions and maintaining healthy actions. It involves an understanding of symptoms, ability to adhere to medication regimens, and knowing when to seek professional medical help/advice.[11,12] Complementary to this are lifestyle modifications that target the behavioral changes required for long-term health enhancement, such as increasing physical activity, managing stress, quitting smoking, and adopting a healthier diet.[13,14] Collectively, these strategies underpin a holistic approach to patient education.

The Crucial Role of Medication Adherence

Medication adherence, the extent to which patients take their medications as prescribed, has been documented as a key factor in effective health care.[15–17] Throughout history, the success of any treatment plan has relied heavily on the patients' willingness and their capacity to follow through with these regimens.[18] This complexity is influenced by such factors as patients understanding of their conditions and treatments, the quality of communication with health care providers, the complexity of the medication schedules themselves, and the strength of support systems accessible to patients.[19,20]

Strengthening Support Through Community and Peer Education

The presence of a robust support system, including family, friends, health care providers, and community resources, can greatly influence a patient's ability to manage their chronic disease.[21] Support systems provide emotional encouragement, practical assistance, and can help reinforce the importance of adherence to treatment plans.[22,23] They act as a safety net, offering reminders for medication schedules, assistance with transportation to health care appointments, and help in understanding and navigating the health care system.[24] Peer education leverages the experiences of individuals who have successfully managed their chronic conditions, to educate and support others facing similar challenges.[25–27] This approach is grounded in the principle that patients can learn effectively from others who have firsthand experience with the same health issues. Peer educators can offer practical advice, emotional support, and motivational encouragement, all of which are essential for long-term disease management.[26]

Objectives of This Article

This article underscores the pivotal role of patient education in the management of chronic diseases. It delves into how educating patients about their conditions, emphasizing the importance of medication adherence, drawing attention to how lifestyle choices that affect disease progression, and leveraging on peer educators and support systems, collectively form the backbone of effective disease management. The goal is to draw attention to how well-informed patients are more likely to adopt self-care habits, identify signs of complications, and actively engage with health care providers consequently leading to better health outcomes.

UNDERSTANDING CHRONIC DISEASES
Definition and Impact

This section examines the definition and impact of chronic diseases. According to the Centers for Disease Control and Prevention, chronic illnesses are broadly defined as conditions that last 1 year or more and require ongoing medical attention or limit activities of daily living or both.[28] These conditions, including prevalent diseases, such as heart disease and cancer, not only lead to significant physiologic and psychosocial challenges but also represent the leading causes of disability and mortality in the United States.[29–31] The financial implications are profound, with chronic disease conditions contributing to the nation's health care costs, which stood at $4.1 trillion in 2023.[32] Beyond the direct medical expenses, chronic diseases significantly reduce the quality of life for individuals and place a considerable economic burden on productivity.[33] This, in turn, presents profound challenges not only to personal finances but also to the economic structure of communities at large.

Role of Patient Education

Patient education is a pivotal element in managing chronic diseases, empowering patients and caregivers with the knowledge, skills, and confidence necessary for effective health management.[34] In chronic heart failure, for example, effective self-management behaviors, such as regular monitoring of weight to detect fluid retention early, adhering to a low-sodium diet to prevent exacerbation of symptoms, engaging in prescribed physical activity to improve cardiovascular health, and taking prescribed medications to manage the condition and prevent hospital readmissions, are encouraged through patient education.[35–37] Furthermore, the personal narratives of patients shared during such educational encounters offer deep insights into the physical and psychological effects of chronic diseases, emphasizing the importance of listening to and learning from patients.[38] This facet of patient education is vital and emphasizes the personalized nature of chronic diseases. Together, these points advocate for a holistic approach that incorporates current information, tailored care, and active involvement from patients.

LIFESTYLE MODIFICATIONS AND SELF-MANAGEMENT

This section explores the multidimensional influence of lifestyle changes (eg, dietary improvements, regular physical activity, stress management techniques, and self-care strategies) in fostering patient empowerment. By delving into the sociocultural, historical, clinical, and pragmatic perspectives of each domain, we illustrate the immense impact of lifestyle changes on patient autonomy and their effectiveness in disease management.

Diet

Historically, the philosophy of "let food be thy medicine" has guided the integration of dietary modifications in the management of chronic diseases. The advent of nutritional science has provided a clinical basis for this approach, emphasizing the need for patient education on the nutritional value of foods, the principles of a balanced diet, and the specific dietary alterations beneficial for their condition.[39] A holistic approach to patient education on nutrition not only encompasses the biologic value of food but also integrates sociocultural beliefs and historical dietary practices to enhance the relevance and acceptance of dietary advice.[40] For example, educating patients on reducing sodium intake to manage hypertension or adopting a diet rich in fiber to combat diabetes should also consider cultural food preferences and historical dietary patterns. This ensures that dietary recommendations are not only clinically effective but also culturally sensitive and practically achievable.

Physical Activity

The prescription of physical activity for disease management is a practice with deep roots in socioclinical history. The Ancient Greeks, for instance, eulogized the virtues of exercise for overall health, a view that has been continuously supported by clinical research over the centuries. In modern medicine, patient education on physical activity goes well beyond the simple of act of moving, jogging, running, or hiking to encompass a broader understanding of its benefits on the physical, emotional, and mental health of patients.[41] This includes practical advice on incorporating activity into daily routines and strategies for overcoming modern-day barriers to maintaining a regular, achievable exercise regimen. Health care professionals can draw from the rich tapestry of historical insights and clinical evidence to craft personalized exercise plans that take into account, the patient's limitations, lifestyle, and preferences.[42]

Stress Management

The challenge of stress management in the context of chronic illness is best addressed by drawing on a wide range of practices, from age-old relaxation techniques to modern theories of psychology. Educating patients about stress management can include not only clinical evidence but also historical sociocultural anecdotes on such techniques as mindfulness, deep breathing, and yoga.[43] By couching these practices within a broader cultural context, patients can appreciate and draw toward their relevance, promoting a more integrated approach to stress management.[44] These not only help in coping with the psychosocial burdens of chronic diseases but also underscores the patient's role in actively managing their care.

Self-Management Strategies

Patient education on self-management strategies represents a synthesis of clinical guidance, personal empowerment, and historical self-care practices. By educating and encouraging patients to monitor symptoms, track medications, and make informed health decisions, health care providers are not just imparting clinical knowledge but are also empowering patients with a sense of agency over their health.[12] Offering such tools as symptom diaries, medication reminders, and decision-making aids not only supports treatment plans but also buttresses principles of self-care and personal health management.

In summary educating patients plays a role in encouraging lifestyle changes and self-management practices in managing diseases. By concentrating on such aspects as diet, exercise, and stress management and empowering patients through education health care professionals can arm individuals with the knowledge and abilities required to handle their conditions. This strategy not only enhances health outcomes but also boosts patients' quality of life thus showcasing the significant impact of patient education on chronic disease management.[45]

MEDICATION ADHERENCE

This section explores the critical role of medication adherence in chronic disease management. Medication adherence just like the other factors discussed is a major determinant of a successful chronic disease management plan. According to Cramer and colleagues, it is defined as "act or extent of conforming to a provider recommendation/prescription based on timing, dosage, and frequency of medication use.[46]" The term is often used interchangeably with medication compliance, although there are divergent views on their usage. Despite the known benefits of medication adherence, many patients struggle to maintain it, leading to suboptimal health outcomes.

Challenges to Adherence

Several factors contribute to poor medication adherence among patients with chronic diseases. These include the following:

- Complex medication regimens: Patients prescribed multiple medications (polypharmacy) with different schedules may find it difficult to remember when and how to take each one.
- Side effect concerns: The fear, perception, or experience of side effects could discourage patients from following their medication regimen.
- Cost: The steep costs associated with medications can pose an obstacle to adherence for individuals lacking sufficient insurance coverage or those in lower income brackets.
- Lack of comprehension: Patients who lack an understanding of their condition or the importance of their medication are less likely to stick to their treatment plan.
- Psychological challenges: Such conditions as depression, anxiety, and other mental health issues can have an impact on a patient's motivation and ability to adhere to their prescribed treatment.

Patient Education Strategies to Improve Medication Adherence

- Simplifying medication schedules: Health care providers should aim to simplify medication regimen whenever feasible making it easier for patients to stick to them.
- Managing side effects: Educating patients on side effects and how to handle them can reduce concerns and boost adherence. Adjusting medications in some instances may be necessary to minimize side effects.
- Financial support: Sharing details about financial aid programs or more affordable medication options can help overcome cost-related barriers to adherence.
- Improving understanding: Providing easy-to-understand information about the medical condition being treated and the significance of each medication in managing it can empower patients to adhere to their treatment plans. This may include using language and visual aids.
- Addressing psychological barriers: Incorporating health support into disease management can assist in tackling psychological hurdles related to medication adherence. This may include counseling, support groups or psychiatric care, for underlying health issues.

Role of Health Care Providers

- Building trusting relationships: A strong patient-provider relationship, characterized by open communication and mutual respect, can significantly enhance adherence. Patients are more likely to follow the advice of providers they trust.

- Personalized education: Tailoring education to the individual patient's needs, beliefs, and preferences can improve understanding and motivation. This includes acknowledging and addressing specific concerns about medication.
- Regular follow-up: Regular check-ins with patients can help providers monitor adherence, address any emerging issues, and adjust treatment plans as necessary.
- Using technology: Digital tools, such as medication reminders via apps or text messages, can support patients in maintaining adherence. Electronic health records can also facilitate the monitoring of prescription refills and adherence patterns.

SUPPORT SYSTEMS AND PEER EDUCATION

This section delves into the significance of support systems and peer education. Patients dealing with illnesses should not face their journey alone. The support from health care providers, family, friends, and caregivers is essential in improving health outcomes and overall well-being. This section delves into the significance of having a support system, the benefits of peer education, and strategies to incorporate support into patient care emphasizing the importance of educating patients and their support network.

Significance of Support Systems

Support systems offer informational and practical help that is necessary for individuals managing chronic conditions. Emotional support assists patients in coping with the effects of their illness, reducing feelings of isolation and depression. Curated informational support provides knowledge and advice that can assist in disease management. Practical assistance, such as aiding with daily tasks or accompanying to appointments, can relieve some burden associated with managing illnesses. The presence of a support system has been associated with enhanced medication adherence, healthier lifestyle choices, and improved disease outcomes.

The Advantages of Peer Education

Peer education involves individuals sharing their experiences, knowledge, and coping mechanisms with others who are encountering similar health issues. This educational approach has benefits, which include the following:

- Enhanced learning: Patients typically find information conveyed by their peers to be more relatable and understandable. Peer educators can simplify complex medical terminology into easier-to-understand language, making health-related information more accessible.
- Boosted motivation: Witnessing friends and family effectively handling their conditions can serve as a source of inspiration and encouragement for patients to embrace habits and stick to treatment plans.
- Emotional support: Peer education fosters a sense of community among patients reducing feelings of isolation by offering a platform for support and motivation.
- Empowerment: Through participation in peer education activities, patients develop confidence in managing their conditions, resulting in increased self-assurance and empowerment.

INTEGRATING SUPPORT IN PATIENT CARE: FOCUS ON EDUCATING SUPPORT SYSTEM/PERSONS

Integrating support systems into patient care requires a concerted effort to educate not only patients but also their families, friends, and caregivers. This approach ensures that the patient's support network is well-informed and equipped to provide the necessary assistance. Strategies for integrating support include the following:

- Inclusive education sessions: Health care providers should offer education sessions that patients can attend with their support persons. These sessions can cover disease information, treatment plans, lifestyle modifications, and strategies for providing support.
- Resources for supporters: Providing written materials, online resources, and access to support groups can help educate and empower the patient's support network.
- Training on specific support tasks: Some patients may require assistance with specific tasks, such as wound care or medication management. Training for family members or caregivers on these tasks ensures that patients receive proper care at home.
- Encouraging open communication: Health care providers should encourage patients and their support persons to communicate openly about their needs, concerns, and preferences. This can help in tailoring support to the patient's individual needs.

THEORETIC FRAMEWORKS

This section explores the theoretic frameworks that underpin patient education in chronic disease management. These frameworks serve as a foundational guide for understanding and influencing patient behaviors. They provide structured approaches and strategies based on psychological and sociologic theories to design educational interventions that encourage patients to engage in their health care and adhere to treatment plans effectively. A condensed exploration of four critical frameworks that shape patient education follows.

- Health Belief Model: This model suggests that a patient's actions are largely driven by personal beliefs about health risks and outcomes.[47] In practical terms, it is about connecting the dots for patients between their condition's severity and the positive impact of adherence. Through Health Belief Model, patient education becomes a tool to shift perceptions, thereby fostering a readiness to embrace healthier behaviors.
- Social Cognitive Theory: Social Cognitive Theory brings to light the power of vicarious experience and self-belief.[48] Witnessing peers successfully manage their health is transformative, providing the confidence needed to take charge of one's own health. Incorporating Social Cognitive Theory into patient education means leveraging success stories and peer-led initiatives to boost individual motivation and self-management skills.
- Chronic Care Model: Chronic Care Model is about establishing a symbiotic ecosystem within health care, where informed patients engage actively with a proactive health care team.[49] Implementing Chronic Care Model involves weaving education into every health care touchpoint, standardizing messages about disease management, and equipping patients with the necessary tools to be proactive participants in their care.
- Motivational Interviewing and Patient Engagement: These concepts stress the significance of patients' active participation in their health care journey.[50] Motivational interviewing, in particular, tailors the educational approach to the patients' readiness to change, addressing any ambivalence and nudging them toward proactive health management. It is about creating an educational

dialogue that resonates with patients wherever they are on their journey to better health.

BEST PRACTICES AND STRATEGIES

This section examines best practices and strategies in patient education for chronic disease management. Adopting evidence-based approaches, leveraging digital health interventions, and implementing practical tips for health care professionals are critical strategies.

Evidence-Based Approaches

Evidence-based approaches in patient education involve using interventions that have been proven effective through rigorous research.[51] These include customized education programs tailored to specific diseases, which have been shown to enhance patient understanding, self-management skills, and adherence to medication regimens.[52] For instance, diabetes self-management education initiatives have demonstrated improvements in glycemic control and reduction in long-term complications. Another effective approach is the use of decision aids, which help patients understand their treatment options and the potential outcomes.

Digital Health Interventions

The incorporation of digital health interventions into patient education offers innovative ways to support chronic disease management. Mobile health applications and software equip patients with tools for monitor symptoms, medications, and physical activity, thereby enhancing their ability to self-manage.[53] Telehealth services facilitate remote consultations, education sessions, and follow-ups, making health care more accessible, especially for those in remote/underserved areas or with mobility issues. Wearable devices enable monitoring of signs and physical activities offering valuable data for patients and health care providers to make informed care decisions. Digital interventions have been particularly effective in increasing engagement and adherence among younger populations, who are generally more tech-savvy.

Practical Tips for Health Care Professionals

For health care professionals, implementing practical tips can significantly enhance the effectiveness of patient education.

- Personalize education: Tailor education to meet each patient's needs, preferences, and learning style. Personalizing the information increases its relevance and engagement making it more likely that patients will remember and apply it in their daily routines.
- Use teach-back method: Implement the teach-back technique to ensure patients grasp the information provided. Asking patients to explain the details in their words can help identify any misunderstandings and offer opportunities for clarification.
- Include visual tools: Integrate aids, such as diagrams, charts, and videos, alongside instructions. Visual tools can simplify information and enhance patient understanding.
- Foster curiosity: Cultivate a supportive atmosphere that encourages patients to ask questions. Addressing inquiries can debunk misconceptions and ease worries. Make it a routine to ensure that patients feel listened to and valued.
- Follow-up: Schedule follow-up appointments or calls to check on patients' progress, address any issues, and reinforce key messages. Regular follow-ups

demonstrate ongoing support and can motivate patients to stay engaged in their care.

CHALLENGES AND CONSIDERATIONS

This section explores the challenges and considerations in effective patient education for chronic disease management. Effective patient education in chronic disease management faces numerous challenges, including issues related to health literacy, access to resources, and cultural competence. Addressing these factors is critical for ensuring that patient education efforts are inclusive, equitable, and effective.

Health Literacy

Health literacy encompasses individuals' capacity to acquire, interpret, and apply essential health information for sound decision-making. The barrier of low health literacy can obstruct a patient's ability to grasp medical concepts, adhere to treatment protocols, or understand the critical role of lifestyle changes. Such barriers often translate into adverse health effects, more frequent hospital admissions, and escalated health care expenses. To address this, health care providers are tasked with distilling complex information into digestible language and confirming patient comprehension, using such strategies as the teach-back method to ensure clarity and understanding.

Resource Accessibility

Ensuring that patients have access to educational and health care resources is pivotal. Those residing in remote areas, individuals with lower socioeconomic status, or those without reliable Internet may face significant challenges in reaching digital health platforms, obtaining educational content, or receiving consistent medical care. This lack of access can widen health disparities and impede efficient disease control. Remedial actions, such as deploying mobile health units, establishing local health initiatives, and providing physical educational tools, are essential to guarantee equitable resource availability for chronic condition management.

Cultural Proficiency

Cultural proficiency in health care is the recognition and respect for diverse cultural distinctions and the delivery of services that are attuned to the cultural needs of individuals. A patient's cultural norms can deeply impact their views on health, illness, and the medical system, influencing their readiness to seek treatment, follow medical advice, and modify lifestyles. Health care workers should aim to become well-versed in the cultural contexts of their patients, tailor care strategies to align with cultural preferences, and use culturally tailored educational resources. Education in cultural proficiency enables health care professionals to identify and navigate cultural obstacles to patient education and involvement effectively.

FUTURE DIRECTIONS AND OPPORTUNITIES

This section provides an overview of future directions and opportunities in patient education for chronic disease management. As the landscape of patient education in chronic disease management continues to evolve, several key areas present promising opportunities for enhancing care and improving patient outcomes. Although a subsequent article delves into these topics in depth, a brief overview highlights the potential of innovations in digital health, personalized medicine, and policy and health care system changes.

Innovations in Digital Health

Advances in digital health is set to transform patient education with the help of artificial intelligence–powered applications, interactive virtual learning experiences, and wearable devices for ongoing health monitoring. These technologies aim to simplify self-management and provide patients with up-to-date information and practical data to support their health care choices.

Personalized Medicine

Personalized medicine, fueled by genomics, heralds a new era of customized patient education and therapy regimens based on individual genetic profiles. This bespoke approach is expected to boost treatment precision, reduce side effects, and actively engage patients by offering treatments specifically suited to their genetic blueprints.

Policy and Health Care System Evolution

Future shifts in policy and health care infrastructure are crucial to facilitate patient education initiatives. Policies geared toward broadening the reach of educational resources, encouraging digital health adoption, and integrating personalized medicine into routine care will be pivotal in enriching chronic disease management. Furthermore, health care systems are transitioning toward more patient-centric models, where education is integral to care delivery.

SUMMARY

The intricate role that patient education plays in managing chronic health conditions has been explored, drawing attention to the need for strategies grounded in solid evidence, digital health solutions, and practical approaches for health care professionals. The article addresses pivotal challenges including the mastery of health literacy, the provision of accessible resources, and the achievement of cultural proficiency, underscoring the critical need for tailored patient-centered approaches. The advent of groundbreaking digital health technologies, the customization of medicine, and shifts in policy frameworks offer alluring prospects for the evolution of patient education.

The conclusions for medical practice are straightforward: impactful patient education is essential for patient empowerment, increased compliance with treatment regimens, and the betterment of overall health metrics. It is imperative for health care providers to give patient education the emphasis it deserves, deploying an assortment of instruments and methodologies to accommodate the varied demands of patients. To optimize the impact of patient education, healthcare providers should focus on several key pearls and be mindful of potential pitfalls.

CLINICS CARE POINTS

Pearls for effective patient education:

- Patient-Centered Education: Tailor educational content to individual patient needs, preferences, and literacy levels to enhance understanding and retention.
- Teach-Back Method: Implement the teach-back technique to confirm patient comprehension, where patients repeat the information in their own words.

- Regular Follow-Up: Schedule follow-up appointments or calls to review progress, answer questions, and reinforce education, ensuring continuous support.
- Cultural Competence: Adapt educational materials and approaches to respect cultural, linguistic, and personal beliefs, ensuring inclusivity and relevance.
- Utilize Family and Caregivers: Involve family members and caregivers in the educational process to extend support networks and enhance adherence.

Pitfalls to avoid in patient education

- Information overload
- Assumptions and misunderstanding
- Inconsistent messaging
- Neglecting emotional aspects
- Understanding barriers

DISCLOSURE

The author declares no commercial or financial conflicts of interest. This work was supported by the National Institute of Minority Health and Health Disparities (NIMHD) under the award number R25 MD007610.

REFERENCES

1. Busse R, Blümel M, Scheller-Kreinsen D, Zentner A. Tackling Chronic Diseases in Europe—Strategies, Interventions and Challenges. In: Observatory Studies Series No 20. Copenhagen: World Health Organization; 2010.
2. Fontana L. From chronic disease to chronic health: the evolving role of doctors in the 21st century. Eur Heart J 2024. https://doi.org/10.1093/eurheartj/ehae173.
3. Hung MJ. Diabetes, hypertension and cardiovascular disease: clinical insights, mechanisms and pharmacotherapies. Medicina 2024;60(4):566.
4. Balakumar P, Maung UK, Jagadeesh G. Prevalence and prevention of cardiovascular disease and diabetes mellitus. Pharmacol Res 2016;113:600–9.
5. Salvi S, Kumar GA, Dhaliwal RS, et al. The burden of chronic respiratory diseases and their heterogeneity across the states of India: the Global Burden of Disease Study 1990–2016. Lancet Global Health 2018;6(12):e1363–74.
6. Geneau R, Stuckler D, Stachenko S, et al. Series chronic diseases: chronic diseases and development 1 Raising the priority of preventing chronic diseases: a political process. Lancet 2010. https://doi.org/10.1016/S0140-6736(10)61414-6.
7. Hattab AS. Healthcare Ethics. In: Laher I, editor. Handbook of healthcare in the Arab World. Springer International Publishing; 2021. p. 1603–19.
8. Haldane V, Jung AS, De Foo C, et al. Strengthening the basics: public health responses to prevent the next pandemic. Br Med J 2021;375. https://doi.org/10.1136/bmj-2021-067510.
9. Dumez V, Pomey M-P. From Medical Paternalism to Care Partnerships: A Logical Evolution Over Several Decades. In: Pomey M-P, Denis J-L, Dumez Vi, editors. Patient Engagement: Organizational Behaviour in Healthcare. Cham: Palgrave Macmillan; 2019. https://doi.org/10.1007/978-3-030-14101-1_2.
10. Jiang Y, Wang W. Health Promotion and Self-Management Among Patients with Chronic Heart Failure. In: Haugan G, Eriksson M, editors. Health Promotion in Health

Care – Vital Theories and Research. Cham: Springer; 2021. https://doi.org/10.1007/978-3-030-63135-2_19.

11. van Beest W, Boon WPC, Andriessen D, et al. Successful implementation of self-management health innovations. J Publ Health 2022;30(3):721–35.

12. Dineen-Griffin S, Garcia-Cardenas V, Williams K, et al. Helping patients help themselves: A systematic review of self-management support strategies in primary health care practice. PLoS One 2019;14(8).

13. Lambrinou E, Hansen TB, Beulens JWJ. Lifestyle factors, self-management and patient empowerment in diabetes care. Eur J Prev Cardiol 2019;26(2_suppl): 55–63.

14. Kim S, Park M, Song R. Effects of self-management programs on behavioral modification among individuals with chronic disease: A systematic review and meta-analysis of randomized trials. PLoS One 2021;16(7 July).

15. Neiman AB, Ruppar T, Michael H, et al. Morbidity and Mortality Weekly Report CDC Grand Rounds: improving medication adherence for chronic disease management-innovations and opportunities innovative strategies to improve medication adherence for chronic disease management. 2017. Available at: https://www.ncpanet.org/pdf/reportcard/AdherenceReportCard.

16. Wilhelmsen NC, Eriksson T. Medication adherence interventions and outcomes: An overview of systematic reviews. Eur J Hosp Pharm 2019;26(4):187–92.

17. Gast A, Mathes T. Medication adherence influencing factors - An (updated) overview of systematic reviews. Syst Rev 2019;8(1).

18. Van Dulmen S, Sluijs E, Van Dijk L, et al. Patient adherence to medical treatment: a review of reviews. BMC Health Serv Res 2007;7. https://doi.org/10.1186/1472-6963-7-55.

19. Kardas P, Lewek P, Matyjaszczyk M. Determinants of patient adherence: a review of systematic reviews. Front Pharmacol 2013. https://doi.org/10.3389/fphar.2013.00091.

20. Dimatteo MR, Giordani PJ, Lepper HS, et al. Patient adherence and medical treatment outcomes a meta-analysis. Care 2002;40(9):794–811.

21. Thompson DM, Booth L, Moore D, et al. Peer support for people with chronic conditions: a systematic review of reviews. BMC Health Serv Res 2022;22(1).

22. Bustamante AV, Vilar-Compte M, Ochoa Lagunas A. Social support and chronic disease management among older adults of Mexican heritage: a U.S.-Mexico perspective. Soc Sci Med 2018;216:107–13.

23. Dinh TTH, Bonner A. Exploring the relationships between health literacy, social support, self-efficacy and self-management in adults with multiple chronic diseases. BMC Health Serv Res 2023;23(1).

24. Korenhof SA, Rouwet EV, Elstgeest LEM, et al. The effect of a community-based group intervention on chronic disease self-management in a vulnerable population. Front Public Health 2023;11. https://doi.org/10.3389/fpubh.2023.1221675.

25. Willis E. Patients' self-efficacy within online health communities: facilitating chronic disease self-management behaviors through peer education. Health Commun 2016;31(3):299–307.

26. Fisher EB, Ballesteros J, Bhushan N, et al. Analysis & commentary: key features of peer support in chronic disease prevention and management. Health Aff 2015; 34(9):1523–30.

27. Embuldeniya G, Veinot P, Bell E, et al. The experience and impact of chronic disease peer support interventions: a qualitative synthesis. Patient Educ Counsel 2013;92(1):3–12.

28. Goodman RA, Posner SF, Huang ES, et al. Defining and measuring chronic conditions: imperatives for research, policy, program, and practice. Prev Chronic Dis 2013;10(4):1–16.

29. Mokdad AH, Ballestros K, Echko M, et al. The State of US Health, 1990-2016. JAMA 2018;319(14):1444.

30. Tinker A. How to improve patient outcomes for chronic diseases and comorbidities. 2017. Available at: http://www.healthcatalyst.com/wp-content/uploads/2014/04/How-to-Improve-Patient-Outcomes.pdf. [Accessed 15 May 2024].

31. Raghupathi W, Raghupathi V. An empirical study of chronic diseases in the United States: a visual analytics approach. Int J Environ Res Publ Health 2018;15(3).

32. Centers for Disease Control and Prevention. Health and Economic Costs of Chronic Diseases. National Center for Chronic Disease Prevention and Health Promotion (NCCDPHP). 2024. Available at: https://www.cdc.gov/chronicdisease/about/costs/index.htm#print. [Accessed 15 May 2024].

33. Fouad AM, Waheed A, Gamal A, et al. Effect of chronic diseases on work productivity. J Occup Environ Med 2017;59(5):480–5.

34. Stoner AM, Cannon M, Shan L, et al. The Other 45: improving patients' chronic disease self-management and medical students' communication skills. J Am Osteopath Assoc 2018;118(11):703–12.

35. Zuraida E, Irwan AM, Sjattar EL. Self-management education programs for patients with heart failure: A literature review. Central European Journal of Nursing and Midwifery 2021;12(1):279–94.

36. Korzh O, Krasnokutskiy S. Significance of education and self-management support for patients with chronic heart failure in family physician practice. Fam Med Prim Care Rev 2016;18(4):432–6.

37. Zeng W, Chia SY, Chan YH, et al. Factors impacting heart failure patients' knowledge of heart disease and self-care management. Proc Singapore Healthc 2017; 26(1):26–34.

38. Brokerhof IM, Ybema JF, Matthijs Bal P. Illness narratives and chronic patients' sustainable employability: the impact of positive work stories. PLoS One 2020;15(2).

39. Hauser ME, McMacken M, Lim A, et al. Nutrition-an evidence-based, practical approach to chronic disease prevention and treatment. J Fam Pract 2022; 71(1):S5–16.

40. Ojo O, Adegboye ARA. The effects of nutrition on chronic conditions. Nutrients 2023;15(5).

41. Haseler C, Crooke R, Haseler T. Promoting physical activity to patients. Med J 2019;366:1–7.

42. Posadzki P, Pieper D, Bajpai R, et al. Exercise/physical activity and health outcomes: an overview of Cochrane systematic reviews. BMC Publ Health 2020;20(1).

43. Tellhed U, Daukantaitė D, Maddux RE, et al. Yogic breathing and mindfulness as stress coping mediate positive health outcomes of Yoga. Mindfulness (N Y) 2019; 10(12):2703–15.

44. Aker A, Serghides L, Cotnam J, et al. The impact of a stress management intervention including cultural components on stress biomarker levels and mental health indicators among indigenous women. J Behav Med 2023;46(4):594–608.

45. Collins C, Rochfort A. Promoting self-management and patient empowerment in primary care." primary care in practice - integration is needed. InTech 2016;11: 28–35.

46. Cramer JA, Roy A, Burrell A, et al. Medication compliance and persistence: terminology and definitions. Value Health 2008;11(1):44–7.

47. Janz NK, Becker MH. The health belief model: a decade later. Health Educ Q 1984;11(1):1–47.
48. Luszczynska A, Schwarzer R. Social cognitive theory. In: Conner M, Norman P, editors. Predicting and changing health behaviour: research and practice with social cognition models. 2015. p. 225–51.
49. Coleman K, Austin BT, Brach C, et al. Evidence on the Chronic Care Model in the new millennium. Health Aff 2009;28(1):75–85.
50. Mccarley P. Patient empowerment and motivational interviewing: engaging patients to self-manage their own care. Nephrol Nurs J 2009;36(4):409–13.
51. Niessen LW, Grijseels EWM, Rutten FFH. The evidence-based approach in health policy and health care delivery. Soc Sci Med 2000;51(6):859–69. Available at: www.elsevier.com/locate/socscimed.
52. Masic I, Miokovic M, Muhamedagic B. Evidence based medicine: new approaches and challenges. Acta Inf Med 2008;16(4):219.
53. Murray E, Hekler EB, Andersson G, et al. Evaluating digital health interventions: key questions and approaches. Am J Prev Med 2016;51(5):843–51.

Enhancing Patient Education in Hospital Settings

Eric C. Nemec, PharmD, MEd[a], Jennie McKown, MSHS, PA-C[b],*

KEYWORDS

- Patient education • Inpatient care • Hospital • Patient discharge
- Evidence-based practices

KEY POINTS

- This article presents a comprehensive overview of evidence-based strategies for optimizing hospital patient education, emphasizing the need for a collaborative, patient-centered approach.
- The purpose of this study is to describe evidence-based strategies to enhance patient education in hospital settings.
- This study mimics an inpatient hospital stay and describes patient education best practices related to admission and preventative measures, hospital stay, and patient discharge.
- It is structured similarly to an inpatient encounter, encompasses best practices, and culminates in a case study.

INTRODUCTION

According to the American Hospital Association, there were over 34 million hospital admissions in the United States in 2023.[1] This statistic is especially sobering considering that being in the hospital has been called "one of the most disempowering situations one can experience in modern society."[2] The Institute of Medicine has recommended that people have the ability to access patient-appropriate medical information and clinical knowledge, which would allow them to be a "source of control" in making health care decisions.[3,4] Within contemporary health care, there has been a paradigm shift from a paternalistic model where decisions were made on behalf of a patient to one that includes shared decision-making and requires patients to be informed.[5] Along with this change in general practice models, there have also been tremendous changes in the health care landscape, leading to changes related to patient education. For example, in the early 1960s, the Physician Assistant/Associate profession did not yet exist, and pharmacists providing medication information to

[a] Sacred Heart University, 5151 Park Avenue, Fairfield, CT 06825, USA; [b] The Johns Hopkins Hospital, 600 North Wolfe Street, Halsted 677, Baltimore, MD 21287, USA
* Corresponding author.
E-mail address: Jmckown1@jhmi.edu

Physician Assist Clin 9 (2024) 541–552
https://doi.org/10.1016/j.cpha.2024.05.006
physicianassistant.theclinics.com
2405-7991/24/© 2024 Elsevier Inc. All rights are reserved, including those for text and data mining, AI training, and similar technologies.

patients would have been considered unethical by the professional code of conduct.[6,7] According to the latest Interprofessional Education Consortium Core Competencies for Interprofessional Collaborative Practice, health care teams should recognize the knowledge of one's role and of other team members' expertise to address individual and population health outcomes.[8] This framework extends to a team-based approach, whereby individual health professionals provide education within their scope of expertise, which could improve health outcomes. However, while each specialty typically practices in a hospital setting, this does not always pan out in clinical practice due to varying practice models.

Patient education aims to promote patient autonomy, improve adherence to treatment plans, enhance patient satisfaction, and ultimately contribute to better health outcomes.[9,10] It is considered a useful intervention for inpatients, with no known adverse effects, that can improve health outcomes across patients with varying health issues.[11] The purpose of this study is to describe evidence-based strategies to enhance patient education in hospital settings. This study mimics an inpatient hospital stay and describes patient education best practices related to admission and preventative measures, hospital stay, and patient discharge.

PATIENT EDUCATION BEST PRACTICES

Patient education and health literacy are related concepts in health care, but they are distinct and serve different purposes. Patient education refers to the process of providing information, instruction, and support to patients to help them make informed decisions about their health, manage their medical conditions, and engage in healthy behaviors. Health literacy is an individual's ability to obtain, understand, and use health information to make informed decisions about their health and navigate the health care system.[12] Effective patient education considers varying levels of health literacy among patients and aims to tailor information and communication to meet the individual's specific needs and abilities.

Multiple organizations, such as the Agency for Healthcare Research and Quality (AHRQ), the Health Care Education Association , and the Centers for Disease Control and Prevention (CDC), provide insight into best practices to provide effective patient education.[13–15] That said, most of these educational best practices (see **Table 1**, for examples) aim to assist the health care professional in ensuring patient comprehension.[16–18] There is an abundance of published studies that seek to quantify the impact of patient education efforts; clinicians should consider conducting a brief review of available literature to ensure there is not a specific work related to your scenario before working to implement a new initiative.

SPECIFIC PATIENT EDUCATION STRATEGIES
Teach-Back

The "teach-back" method is a patient education technique where health care providers ask patients to repeat information in their own words, ensuring understanding and effective communication. This process starts with the provider explaining a concept clearly, followed by the patient's repetition to confirm comprehension. If misunderstandings are identified, the provider re-explains as needed, using simple language and possibly visual aids. This nonjudgmental, supportive approach encourages patient engagement and clarifies any confusion. Particularly useful for instructions about medications, procedures, or lifestyle changes, teach-back verifies patient understanding and reinforces critical information, significantly improving adherence to care plans and overall health outcomes. "Always use teach-back" is

Table 1 Agency for Healthcare Research and Quality health literacy universal precautions toolkit highlights	
Use the Teach-Back Method	The teach-back strategy entails assessing comprehension by prompting patients to express in their own words the information or steps necessary for managing their health. This method serves as a means to affirm that you have conveyed the information to your patients in a way that they comprehend.
Communicate Clearly	Implementing clear verbal communication strategies can improve patients' grasp of health-related information. Furthermore, clear communication fosters a sense of active involvement in their health care and enhances the likelihood of them adhering to their treatment plans.
Follow Up with Patients	Follow-up involves getting in touch with a patient or caregiver on a scheduled, later date to review the patient's progress since their last appointment.
Consider Culture, Customs, and Beliefs	Religion, culture, individual beliefs, and ethnic customs can play a significant role in shaping how patients perceive health concepts, manage their well-being, and make decisions related to their health care.
Make Action Plans	An action plan, jointly developed by the patient and clinician, delineates straightforward steps that a patient can adopt to reach a health goal, whether it involves weight loss or enhancing their management of a chronic condition.
Help Patients Remember How and When to Take Their Medicine	Research findings have demonstrated that patients frequently encounter challenges in understanding how and when to take their medications, especially when their treatment plans are complicated. Offering support to help patients grasp which medicines they need and the correct administration procedures can significantly reduce medication errors.

an important component of the Institute for Healthcare Improvement's recommended discharge process.[19]

Chunk and Check

The "chunk and check" patient education method simplifies complex medical information into smaller, more manageable segments or "chunks" for easier patient comprehension. This approach involves first breaking down the information into these chunks and then presenting each segment individually. After each chunk is delivered, the health care provider checks the patient's understanding, often by asking them to summarize the information in their own words or by addressing any questions. This checking can be done through various methods, such as asking the patient to summarize the information in their own words, known as the "Teach Back" method, or by observing the patient's nonverbal responses. This cycle is repeated for each piece of information, ensuring the patient fully grasps each concept before moving to the next. Finally, a comprehensive review is conducted, often with a follow-up to reinforce learning and address further queries. This method is particularly effective for improving patient understanding and retention, especially in stressful or overwhelming health care environments.[20]

Show-Me Method

The "show-me" method in patient education is an interactive and practical approach emphasizing hands-on learning. Health care providers demonstrate a task to the patient, such as using an inhaler, and then ask the patient to replicate the action. This active participation allows the patient to practice the skill under supervision, ensuring they understand and can properly perform the necessary procedures for their care. It is a technique that helps retain information and empowers patients by directly involving them in their health care process. This method is particularly beneficial for those who learn better by doing rather than by listening or reading.[13]

HOSPITAL SETTING PATIENT EDUCATION
Inpatient Safety and Preventing Hospital-Acquired Infections

Proper hand hygiene is one of the most effective measures to prevent the spread of infections in health care settings. Patients who maintain good hand hygiene are less likely to acquire infections during their hospital stay, which can lead to improved health outcomes. Teaching patients about hand hygiene encourages active participation in infection prevention, while it is a seemingly simple intervention, it positions them as partners in maintaining a hygienic health care environment. Patients who comprehend the importance of hand hygiene may also be more inclined to advocate for its adherence among health care providers and visitors. This cultural shift promotes mutual respect and an unwavering commitment to patient safety.[21]

Inappropriate antibiotic use has contributed to the public health emergency of antibiotic-resistant organisms.[22] Patient expectation of an antibiotic prescription increases the likelihood of receiving it, even when inappropriate, by as much as 10 fold.[23] The CDC has developed a program entitled Be Antibiotics Aware, a national effort to help fight antibiotic resistance and improve antibiotic prescribing and use. This program contains printable patient education materials to help prescribers educate patients when an antibiotic is an inappropriate therapeutic option, antibiotic resistance, and adverse effects.[23] Educated patients can contribute to antibiotic stewardship by advocating for responsible antibiotic use and recognizing the importance of addressing antibiotic resistance as a global health concern.[24]

Preparing Patients for Procedures and Surgery

The demand to reduce hospital costs, improve quality measures, and reduce hospital length of stay has led to an increasing number of procedures and surgeries being performed in the outpatient setting and accelerated recovery pathways, such as enhanced recovery after surgery (ERAS) programs.[25] ERAS programs are "multidisciplinary care pathways that standardize and optimize perioperative care to improve postoperative outcomes." The main goals of ERAS pathways include reduced length of stay, quicker overall functional recovery, and decreased postoperative nausea, vomiting, and pain.[26]

Whether a procedure is an accelerated recovery pathway or a traditional pathway, patients undergoing an outpatient procedure, or surgery requiring hospital admission, require clear preoperative instructions, including dietary restrictions, medication changes, skin preparation, and other specific adjustments to their normal routine. They may need to prepare for absence from home or work and understand what their recovery may look like. They may have anticipated activity restrictions, bathing or showering restrictions, or require special equipment or support. The health care team should communicate these expectations to the patient before the planned procedure or surgery.

Informed consent is a process of communication between a clinician and a patient that results in the patient being able to make an informed decision regarding whether they want to undergo a procedure or surgery that has been recommended.[27] The informed consent process is one of many opportunities to educate the patient about the planned procedure, explain the benefits and risks of the procedure, and offer alternatives. Often, informed consent is obtained close to the time of the procedure or on the same day of the procedure. Patients may be stressed, tired, anxious, or scared, limiting their ability to comprehend the information fully. It is not uncommon for patients to sign a consent form without fully understanding their options, benefits, and risks.[27]

Prior to the procedure or admission, preoperative information should be discussed with the patient, including what to expect after the procedure or surgery. For example, if incision or wound care is expected, questions that should be considered include the following: will the patient be able to perform wound or incision care themselves, or should they identify someone who can help them? Will the patient be able to walk or drive after the procedure? Will they need help with transportation to appointments? Will they require additional assistance for activities of daily living due to lifting or mobility restrictions? The patient should identify whom they would like the care team to discuss their health with before the procedure or admission. Reviews of the literature have shown that discharge education should begin as soon as the patient is informed of the surgery and should continue throughout the hospitalization period.[28] Some teams provide an example of standardized discharge instructions for review prior to planned procedures. However, care should always be taken to individualize instructions for each patient prior to discharge.[27]

AHRQ offers training modules to health care facilities for health care professionals and leaders to improve the informed consent process. The training modules, called Making Informed Consent an Informed Choice, *help providers communicate clearly, present choices, and help* individuals make informed choices.[29]

Most postoperative complications occur within 30 days after surgery, with up to 1 in 7 surgical patients readmitted within 30 days of a major operation.[30] For many patients undergoing surgery, their ability to manage their own postoperative care is altered due to pain, fatigue, or the presence of wounds, drains, or intravenous lines.[28] Common reasons for readmission include infections, inadequate pain control, gastrointestinal complaints, and failure to thrive. Education efforts often focus on mitigating these complications; however, it is only one component of appropriate follow-up and patient care.

DISCHARGE EDUCATION AND SELF-CARE

A hospital stay can be a significant experience for a patient, and they might encounter several changes or challenges after being discharged. These can vary depending on the reason for hospitalization and the individual's overall health. However, some common things that might be new for a patient after a hospital stay include the diagnosis of a new condition, new medications, self-management skills, and often the need for multiple follow-up appointments. Considering the potential amount of new information, education and teaching should start at the beginning of the hospital stay, recognizing that several teaching sessions may be needed for the patient or family to understand the information or skills being taught fully.[19] Patient education should be a continual process throughout the hospitalization, emphasizing the transition to home and self-care as the discharge date approaches. The discharge date can be difficult to predict accurately and can lead to the delivery of important and large amounts of information on the day of discharge.[31] Discharge education should be adjusted to the individual patient, considering their understanding of their condition and ability to comprehend the material being presented.

Providers should recognize that it can be difficult for patients to navigate the health care system and incorporate strategies to make it easier for patients and families. Making follow-up appointments and filling prescriptions prior to discharge are ways to ease some of the challenges that patients often face when transitioning to home.[19] Having discharge medications at the bedside while reviewing discharge instructions can help with understanding and medication compliance. Ensuring the patient and family have the necessary equipment at home and any requisite home care services are arranged before discharge can help avoid patient safety events at home, such as falls. The discharging team should promptly send the discharge summary, including patient instructions, to the patient's outpatient clinicians, home care team, or nursing or rehab facility so they do not have to rely on the patient for this important information.[19]

Many resources are available for clinicians to help improve the discharge process. For example, Project Re-engineered Discharge (Project RED) is a research group at Boston University Medical Center that focuses on research to improve the hospital discharge process. Project RED has shown that preparing patients to care for themselves upon discharge from the hospital can reduce rehospitalization rates and improve patient safety. The RED toolkit, available on the AHRQ Web site, includes 5 tools that provide step-by-step instructions for implementation. The toolkit addresses language barriers, cross-cultural issues, and disparities in health care communication and trust.[32]

Preventing Hospital Readmissions

Early hospital readmissions (≤30 days following discharge, also known as 30 day readmits) were initially proposed as an indicator of quality of care in the 1980s and have since been used as a quality metric by Medicare and the Department of Veterans Affairs.[33] While the degree to which readmissions are preventable has been a point of debate, patient education plays a vital role in preventing hospital readmissions by equipping patients with the knowledge and skills to manage their health effectively after discharge.[34] Health literacy is not routinely evaluated or recorded in patients' medical records and administrative data; however, patients with lower health literacy are more likely to revisit the emergency room within 90 days of hospital discharge.[35] A recent study suggests that consistently providing more of the recommended evidence-based transitional care processes, including predischarge patient education, may reduce readmissions.[33]

The Hospital Readmissions Reduction Program (HRRP) is a Medicare value-based purchasing program that encourages hospitals to improve communication and care coordination to engage patients and caregivers in discharge plans and, in turn, reduce avoidable readmissions.[36] HRRP focuses on specific medical conditions, including heart failure, acute myocardial infarction (heart attack), pneumonia, chronic obstructive pulmonary disease, elective total hip arthroplasty, and elective total knee arthroplasty. Effective patient education is a key strategy for achieving the HRRP goals while ensuring patients receive the appropriate care they need during and after their hospital stay. Most literature surrounding initiatives focuses on a specific disease state; however, data suggest that medication education can improve outcomes.[37]

Medication Education

While there are many changes upon discharge, new or adjusted medications are often a new or updated part of a patient's lifelong health. Medication counseling before hospital discharge is often proposed as an important component of seamless care. Various clinicians provide counseling; however, in most published studies, pharmacists, nurses, and physicians perform medication counseling at hospital discharge.[38] A systematic literature review found that outcomes were more likely to be significant when assessing medication knowledge and adherence.[38] Educational interventions that are personalized, repeated, and initiated at the time of new disease diagnosis have shown modest success in improving adherence.[39] In practice, providing timely and sustained interventions within the clinical workflow may be challenging. Despite these promising outcomes and the requisite knowledge necessary to engage a patient as their advocate, it remains complex to prove the impact of pharmaceutical care interventions on hospital readmissions, emergency department visits, and mortality.[40,41]

DISCUSSION
Challenges and Considerations

Many early patient education programs emphasized the simple transfer of knowledge related to health status; unfortunately, this does not account for the more complex aspects of health behavior or the ability of a patient to comprehend information.[11] As a result, most early interventions were only effective among the most educated and economically advantaged in the community, as adults with higher levels of education tend to live healthier and longer lives.[11,42,43]

The "Health Literacy Universal Precautions Toolkit" is designed to help primary care practices reduce the complexity of health care, increase patient understanding of health information, and enhance support for patients of all health literacy levels.[13,44] Knowledge is power, and knowledge regarding one's own health should be empowering to the patient. There is not a one-size-fits-all approach to patient education; however, the authors plan to close this study with some tips for success (**Table 2**) as you continue to work to educate your patients.

SUMMARY

Patient education has the potential to improve the patient's understanding and self-management of health conditions, hopefully leading to enhanced patient engagement, which in turn could improve health outcomes. While some literature may conflict with these ideals, patient education remains a cornerstone of quality health care, leading to better patient outcomes, reduced costs, and a more empowered, healthier population.

PATIENT EDUCATION CASE STUDY

A 62 year old patient with type II diabetes mellitus presents to the emergency department with an ulcer on the plantar aspect of the foot with exposed bone that has been present for 4 weeks. There is purulent drainage, surrounding erythema, and tunneling

Table 2	
Patient education tips for success	
Do's	Do Not's
Be clear and concise in your communication	Do not use complicated medical words or abbreviations when you speak or in written material
Use the teach-back method to confirm your patient understands the procedure or their medical situation/diagnosis	Avoid asking "yes" or "no" questions when assessing the patient's understanding
Include patient education with each patient encounter throughout the hospitalization	Do not wait until the day of discharge to begin educating the patient and family
Tailor your approach to the individual patient and how they learn best	Do not provide all the information at once without pausing to make sure the patient understands and is keeping up
Include the patient in planning and decision-making	Refrain from relying solely on the nursing staff to educate your patients. Patient education is most effective as a team approach
Ensure the patient has adequate follow-up appointments and understands their importance	Do not assume that the patients will call and make all their own appointments
Ensure the patient has all the appropriate phone numbers or contact information if questions or concerns arise after discharge. Specify what symptoms should prompt a call to the clinical team	Do not rely on the patient to know when or who to call when questions or problems occur after discharge

of the wound. Point of care Hemoglobin A1C is 10%. Radiograph shows changes consistent with osteomyelitis in the affected foot. The patient does not have palpable pedal pulses. The ankle–brachial index shows noncompressible vessels and a toe pressure of 30 mm Hg on the affected side. A surgery consult is performed. The patient requires admission to the hospital for intravenous antibiotics and surgical debridement.

Patient Education Prior to Admission

Discuss the treatment plan with the patient and their support person or care partner. Confirm that the patient's home medication list is up to date and accurate. Use the teach-back method to confirm that the patient understands the plan of care.

Teach-back method: "We have just covered a lot of information, and I would like to make sure that you understand what I explained. Can you please describe the plan of treatment for your foot wound and infection in your own words?" Remember, nonverbal communication is also important. Comfortable body language and eye contact help the patient feel cared for.

If the patient cannot explain the plan of care in their own words, the provider should re-explain the plan differently so that the patient can understand.

Hospital Course

The patient is admitted and started on broad-spectrum antibiotics for a diabetic foot infection. He undergoes a lower extremity angiogram with angioplasty and stent placement to improve perfusion to his foot to help wound healing. He has serial debridements to remove infected and unhealthy tissue. He is given special footwear to offload the area of incision and wound. A peripherally inserted central catheter (PICC) is placed for 6 weeks of intravenous antibiotic administration for osteomyelitis. He is discharged on long-acting, nutritional, and sliding-scale subcutaneous insulin for glucose control, which is new for him. He is ready to be discharged home 10 days after he was admitted.

In Hospital Education

Every encounter with a patient is an opportunity to educate. If the patient can participate in dressing changes, encourage this and teach and reinforce hand hygiene principles. With each point-of-care glucose test and administration of insulin, the patient can be taught how to perform the test, interpret the results, and appropriate use of basal, nutritional, and sliding-scale insulin.

Discharge Education

The patient's discharge plan will include many significant aspects to consider, including activity restrictions, wound care, and medication administration, including insulin administration and intravenous antibiotics.

Chunk and Check

While reviewing the discharge instructions with the patient and support person, stop frequently and use the teach-back method to ensure the patient understands. If they do not understand, then explain the material again but in a different way.

Handouts

Consider using the PEMAT toolkit from AHRQ to assess patient education materials, including handouts, to evaluate whether patients can understand and act on the information provided. During discharge education, utilize handouts and allow the patient to reference them during teach-back; however, they should not read directly from the handout.

Show-Me Method

To facilitate teaching the patient how to use insulin, have the patient self-administer during their hospitalization. The show-me method can also be utilized to check blood sugar with a glucometer. This patient or caregiver can also demonstrate how to flush the PICC line and perform the recommended dressing change for the foot wound.

CLINICS CARE POINTS

- The landscape of patient education within hospital settings is undergoing a crucial transformation to enhance patient outcomes and empowerment.
- A primary objective of patient education is to empower patients, enabling them to become active participants in their care and shared decision-makers in their health care journey.
- There is a critical distinction between patient education and health literacy, and it underscores the necessity of tailoring educational efforts to individual health literacy levels and introduces best practices for effective patient education, drawing insights from leading health care organizations.

DISCLOSURE

The authors declare no competing interests.

REFERENCES

1. Fast facts on U.S. hospitals, 2023 | AHA. Available at: https://www.aha.org/statistics/fast-facts-us-hospitals. [Accessed 21 November 2023].
2. Bickmore T, Pfeifer L, Jack B. Taking the time to care: Empowering low health literacy hospital patients with virtual nurse agents. Proceedings of the SIGCHI Conference on Human Factors in Computing Systems 2009;1265–74. https://doi.org/10.1145/1518701.1518891.
3. Prey JE, Woollen J, Wilcox L, et al. Patient engagement in the inpatient setting: A systematic review. J Am Med Inform Assoc 2014;21(4):742–50.
4. Tang PC, Lansky D. The missing link: Bridging the patient-provider health information gap. Health Aff (Millwood) 2005;24(5):1290–5.
5. Tran D, Angelos P. How should shared decision making be taught? AMA J Ethics 2020;22(5):388.
6. Urick BY, Meggs EV. Towards a greater professional standing: Evolution of pharmacy practice and education, 1920–2020. Pharmacy (Basel) 2019;7(3):98.
7. Cawley JF, Cawthon E, Hooker RS. Origins of the physician assistant movement in the United States. JAAPA 2012;25(12):36–40, 42.
8. Interprofessional Education Collaborative. IPEC core competencies for interprofessional collaborative practice. 3edition. Washington, DC: Interprofessional Education Collaborative; 2023.
9. Agency for Healthcare Research and Quality. Patient education and engagement. Available at: https://www.ahrq.gov/health-literacy/patient-education/index.html. [Accessed 21 November 2023].
10. Krist AH, Tong ST, Aycock RA, et al. Engaging patients in decision-making and behavior change to promote prevention. Stud Health Technol Inform 2017;240:284–302.
11. Simonsmeier BA, Flaig M, Simacek T, et al. What sixty years of research says about the effectiveness of patient education on health: A second order meta-analysis. Health Psychol Rev 2022;16(3):450–74.
12. Centers for Disease Control and Prevention. What is health literacy?. 2023. Available at: https://www.cdc.gov/healthliteracy/learn/index.html. [Accessed 22 December 2023].
13. AHRQ health literacy universal precautions toolkit 2nd edition. 2020. Available at: https://www.ahrq.gov/health-literacy/improve/precautions/index.html. [Accessed 22 December 2023].
14. Healthcare Education Association. Patient education practice guidelines for health care professionals. Available at: https://www.hcea-info.org/patient-education-practice-guidelines-for-health-care-professionals. [Accessed 22 December 2023].
15. Educating patients. Available at: https://www.cdc.gov/vaccines/hcp/patient-ed/educating-patients.html. [Accessed 22 December 2023].
16. Laws MB, Lee Y, Taubin T, et al. Factors associated with patient recall of key information in ambulatory specialty care visits: Results of an innovative methodology. PLoS One 2018;13(2):e0191940.
17. Tao Y, Liu T, Hua Y, et al. Effects of a temporal self-regulation theory-based intervention on self-management in hemodialysis patients: A randomized controlled trial. Patient Educ Couns 2023;119:108059.
18. Janik F, Fabre C, Seichepine AL, et al. Middle-term effects of education programme in chronic low back pain patients to an adherence to physical activity: A randomized controlled trial. Patient Educ Couns 2023;119:108081.

19. Glick AF, Brach C, Yin HS, et al. Health literacy in the inpatient setting. Pediatr Clin 2019;66(4):805–26.
20. The Health Literacy Place. Chunk and check. Available at: https://www.healt hliteracyplace.org.uk/toolkit/techniques/chunk-and-check/. [Accessed 21 December 2023].
21. McGuckin M, Taylor A, Martin V, et al. Evaluation of a patient education model for increasing hand hygiene compliance in an inpatient rehabilitation unit. Am J Infect Control 2004;32(4):235–8.
22. Lushniak BD. Surgeon general's perspectives. Public Health Rep (1974) 2014; 129(4):314–6.
23. Sirota M, Round T, Samaranayaka S, et al. Expectations for antibiotics increase their prescribing: Causal evidence about localized impact. Health Psychol 2017;36(4):402–9.
24. Miller BJ, Carson KA, Keller S. Educating patients on unnecessary antibiotics: Personalizing potential harm aids patient understanding. J Am Board Fam Med 2020;33(6):969–77.
25. Kang E, Gillespie BM, Tobiano G, et al. General surgical patients' experience of hospital discharge education: A qualitative study. J Clin Nurs 2020;29(1–2). https://doi.org/10.1111/jocn.15057.
26. Afonso AM, Mccormick PJ, Assel MJ, et al. Enhanced recovery programs in an ambulatory surgical oncology center. Anesth Analg 2021;133(6):1391.
27. Shoemaker SJ, Brach C, Edwards A, et al. Opportunities to improve informed consent with AHRQ training modules. Joint Comm J Qual Patient Saf 2018; 44(6):343.
28. Kang E, Gillespie BM, Tobiano G, et al. Discharge education delivered to general surgical patients in their management of recovery post discharge: A systematic mixed studies review. Int J Nurs Stud 2018;87:1–13.
29. Agency for Healthcare Research and Quality. AHRQ's making informed consent an informed choice: Training modules for health care leaders and professionals. 2023. Available at: https://www.ahrq.gov/health-literacy/professional-training/ informed-choice.html. [Accessed 22 December 2023].
30. Jones CE, Hollis RH, Wahl TS, et al. Transitional care interventions and hospital readmissions in surgical populations: A systematic review. Am J Surg 2016; 212(2):327–35.
31. Bajorek SA, McElroy V. Discharge planning and transitions of care. 2020. Available at: https://psnet.ahrq.gov/primer/discharge-planning-and-transitions-care. [Accessed 17 April 2024].
32. Re-Engineered Discharge (RED) Toolkit. Agency for Healthcare Research and Quality. 2023. Available at: https://www.ahrq.gov/patient-safety/settings/hospital/ red/toolkit/index.html. [Accessed 17 April 2024].
33. Pugh J, Penney LS, Noël PH, et al. Evidence based processes to prevent readmissions: More is better, a ten-site observational study. BMC Health Serv Res 2021;21(1):189.
34. van Walraven C, Bennett C, Jennings A, et al. Proportion of hospital readmissions deemed avoidable: A systematic review. Canadian Medical Association Journal (CMAJ) 2011;183(7):E391–402.
35. Shahid R, Shoker M, Chu LM, et al. Impact of low health literacy on patients' health outcomes: A multicenter cohort study. BMC Health Serv Res 2022;22(1): 1–1148.

36. Hospital readmissions reduction program (HRRP). 2023. Available at: https://www.cms.gov/medicare/quality/value-based-programs/hospital-readmissions. [Accessed 7 December 2023].
37. Mills AA, Rodeffer KM, Quick SL. Impact of heart failure transitions of care program: A prospective study of heart failure education and patient satisfaction. Hosp Pharm 2021;56(4):252–8.
38. Capiau A, Foubert K, Van der Linden L, et al. Medication counselling in older patients prior to hospital discharge: A systematic review. Drugs Aging 2020;37(9):635–55.
39. Kini V, Ho PM. Interventions to improve medication adherence: A review. JAMA 2018;320(23):2461–73.
40. Polster D. Preventing readmissions with discharge education. Nurs Manag 2015;46(10):30–7.
41. Non LR. All aboard the ChatGPT steamroller: Top 10 ways to make artificial intelligence work for healthcare professionals. Antimicrob Steward Healthc Epidemiol 2023 Dec 18;3(1):e243.
42. Hoving C, Visser A, Mullen PD, et al. A history of patient education by health professionals in Europe and North America: From authority to shared decision making education. Patient Educ Couns 2010;78(3):275–81.
43. Zajacova A, Lawrence EM. The relationship between education and health: Reducing disparities through a contextual approach. Annu Rev Public Health 2018;39:273–89.
44. Rural Health Information Hub. Stigma of low health literacy. Available at: https://www.ruralhealthinfo.org/toolkits/health-literacy/4/stigma. [Accessed 21 December 2023].

Patient Education for Preventative Health Care

Sarah Schuur, PA-C, MPAS[a],*, Brittany Stokes-Francis, PA-C, MS[b]

KEYWORDS

- Preventative medicine • Clinician-centered care • Patient-centered care
- Health literacy • Health belief model • Diffusion of innovation model
- Self-efficacy theory

KEY POINTS

- Preventative medicine involves efforts toward the prevention of disease for managing the welfare of a health community.
- Preventative medicine remains a challenge in the current health care environment.
- Implementation of effective strategies in patient education pertaining to preventative medicine to enhance health outcomes, reduce costs, enhance patient experience while enhancing quality and safety.
- Evidence-based approaches to patient education within preventative medicine include team-based care, patient-centered care, supporting health literacy, and the use of technology.
- Theoretic frameworks pertinent to patient education focused on prevention include the Health Belief Model, the Diffusion of Innovation Model, and the Self-Efficacy Model.

INTRODUCTION
Overview

In 1736, Benjamin Franklin proclaimed to the Philadelphia colony threatened by a great fire that "An ounce of prevention is worth a pound of cure."[1] This preventative approach to medicine has been coined as the cornerstone of health care. However, effective patient education for preventative health care remains a challenge. It is essential that health care professionals develop skills and competencies on how to provide effective patient education to enhance health outcomes, improve patient experience, reduce costs while enhancing quality and safety.[2] This article presents the current evidence-based practices on patient education for preventative health care. The article summarizes historical trends, theoretic frameworks, and provides tools for the clinician.

[a] Physician Assistant Leadership and Learning Academy, Graduate School, University of Maryland, Baltimore, 520 West Fayette Street, Suite # 130, Baltimore, MD 21201, USA;
[b] Physician Assistant Department, Howard University, 801 North Capitol Street Northeast, Washington, DC 20002, USA
* Corresponding author.
E-mail address: sporterschuur@umaryland.edu

Physician Assist Clin 9 (2024) 553–566
https://doi.org/10.1016/j.cpha.2024.05.007
2405-7991/24/© 2024 Elsevier Inc. All rights are reserved, including those for text and data mining, AI training, and similar technologies.
physicianassistant.theclinics.com

Objectives

After reading this article, clinicians will be able to do the following.

1. Examine the historical development of preventative medicine, emphasizing key milestones, practices, and influential figures.
2. Analyze the differences between patient-centered and provider-centered medical care models, elucidating their respective advantages, disadvantages, and impact on patient engagement and empowerment in preventative medicine.
3. Evaluate key patient education models, such as the Health Belief Model (HBM), the Diffusion of Innovation Model, and the Self-Efficacy Model, with respect to preventative health care settings to understand their theoretic foundations, practical applications, and effectiveness in encouraging preventive health care behavior.
4. Provide patient education within preventative medicine utilizing evidence-based best practices and strategies.
5. Identify the challenges, barriers, and opportunities for improvement in preventative patient education.

Key Concepts

- Patient-Centered Care versus Clinician-Centered Care
- Health Belief Model
- Diffusion of Innovation Model
- Self-Efficacy Model
- Health Literacy

BACKGROUND AND CONTEXT
Historical Perspective

Preventative medicine is a valuable component of patient care. It includes all efforts toward the prevention of disease and is an invaluable tool for managing the welfare of the health community. Envisioning a medical culture in which preventative medicine is not included would be challenging for most health care professionals. However, preventative medicine is a fairly recent concept in medicine.[2]

Although the application of preventative medicine is fairly recent, there are foundations of preventative medicine in ancient Greece.[3] The 5th century Greek physician Hippocrates identified seasonal, climate, and external conditions that were linked to disease. He noted causes such as diet, exercise, and other exposures of the population to health outcomes.[4] These principles of disease prevention were not expanded on leading to generations of poorly managed epidemics that include leprosy and plague.[2] In 1854, Dr John Snow successfully traced the source of London's cholera epidemic to the infamous Broad Street Pump. This information helped to end the epidemic when the pump was decommissioned. Following his success, Dr Snow and his colleagues were among the first to endorse preventive medicine instruction in medical schools.[4] Within the next centuries, growth of scientific knowledge including the development of vaccinations, insulin, and the x-ray, encouraged a global formation and implementation of preventative medicine.[2]

Current Landscape

Preventative medicine had clearly shown its value. However, the early 20th century physicians, trained in apprenticeships as generalists, lacked the formal training for standardized application.

Historical approaches to the management of patients were typically provider-centered, symptom-focused approach in which the medical provider takes charge of the interaction to identify and prevent disease.[5] The clinician would act in the best interest of their patient independently of their patient. Patients were only given information deemed to be needed to persuade them to permit testing or vaccination on an individual and global level.[6] The 1950 Polio mass vaccination campaign is an example. The government authorized national immunization days, sub-national immunization days and "mop-up activities" to ensure the highest possible coverage in the shortest possible time.[6] In many ways, the perspective of health care professionals as expert medical facilitators in a standard clinician-centered model aided in the global acceptance of these efforts.

In modern society, clinician-centered approaches to preventative medicine have not been as successful. Evident by the 2020 coronavirus disease 2019 pandemic, despite a similar approach to public messaging, the coronavirus vaccine was met with hesitancy when compared to the polio vaccine, potentially impacted by technological advances of social media and medical messaging.[7] Organizational team-based efforts including the Kaiser Permanente, the California Department of Health, and the California Coronavirus Testing Task Force utilize community outreach, and social media to create resources to educate unimmunized populations.[8] Clinical providers are uniquely suited to take leadership roles providing patient-centered care focusing on facilitating knowledge, attitudes, and skills necessary to maintain or improve health.[9] See (**Fig. 1**) for more information regarding clinician-centered versus patient-centered care.

Theoretic Foundations

a. Theoretic Frameworks (**Fig. 2**)
b. Application to Patient Education

The Health Belief Model

Developed in the 1950s by the United States Public Health Service, the HBM was formulated to explain preventive health behavior.[10] The creation of HBM was in response to a low number of persons being screened for tuberculosis despite efforts to make screening available. Humans are more complicated, and their behavior is more challenging to activate than simply applying positive and negative reinforcements.[10] The ability for people to apply reasoning to their decision making needed to be addressed. A person's behavior reflects the value and desirability of and outcome.

The HBM recognizes the value of avoiding illness utilizing the expectation that certain behaviors may aid in prevention or treatment.[10,11] It suggests that health care recommendations will have the largest patient population impact by targeting perceived barriers, benefits, self-efficacy, and threat. The HBM suggests that there are 6 predictors of health behavior. They are: (1) risk susceptibility, (2) risk severity, (3) benefits to action, (4) barriers to action, (5) self-efficacy, and (6) cues to action.[11]

To optimally apply this theory, patient education must consider the aforementioned variables. The intent of the HBM is to increase self-efficacy. By creating an efficacy-centered message, the health provider or institution hope that increased perceptions of self-efficacy will encourage the patient to recognize the benefits of engaging in the behavior.[11] See **Fig. 3** for an example of the HBM.

Diffusion of innovation model

The Diffusion of Innovation Theory (DOI) was first theorized in the early 20th century. In 1936, Ralph Linton wrote, "Diffusion really includes 3 fairly distinct processes: presentation of the new culture element or elements to the society, acceptance by the

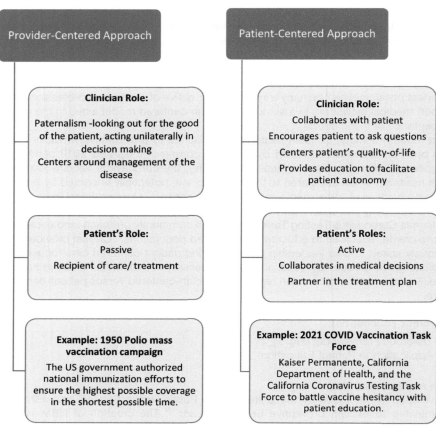

Fig. 1. Clinician-centered vs patient-centered approach.[5,6,8]

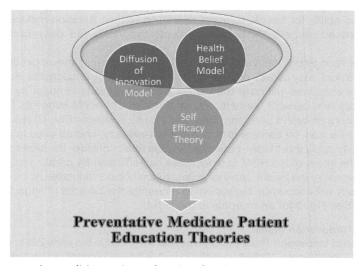

Fig. 2. Preventative medicine patient education theories.

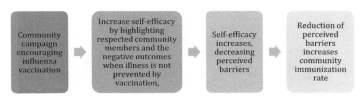

Fig. 3. Example of the Health Belief Model (HBM).

society, and the integration of the accepted element or elements into the preexisting culture."[12]

The concept of the DOI theory can be divided into 2 parts: innovation and diffusion. "Diffusion" is the process by which a new concept is shared within a specific period. By the 1950s, diffusion researchers had begun to apply the collective knowledge to predict and influence the spread of health-related concepts and recommendations.[12] This theory observed that successful, effective practices and programs frequently do not achieve the desired impact therefore failing mediate a poor outcome for residents, clients, patients, and other populations at risk.[12] The resulting dissemination science is the studies the best techniques to communicate evidence-based practices, programs, and policies.

"Innovation," the second part of the DOI theory, refers to the new concept that will be diffused in the population. Innovations include practices, products, services, or devices useful to a specific population.[13] The DOI recognizes that innovation does not end with the identification of a novel idea. The innovation must then be adopted, and practitioners need the ability to change attitudes and behavior of the desired population.[12,13] An example of putting the DOI into practice is through use of online social networks. In the communication of information through online social networks, individuals can disseminate innovativeness to a desired population to reach a certain level of awareness.[13]

When educating a patient on preventative medicine recommendations, it can be challenging to explain the value of illness prevention. Medical providers may be frustrated by unsupported medical information online that may cause the patient to question the value and risk of a preventative intervention.

The DOI theory encourages the application of high-technology media to provide evidence-based guidance. With rapid transmission of reliable tools to educate patients, health care professionals are able to meet the demand of health needs, such as vaccine education (**Fig. 4**).[13]

Self-efficacy theory

Self-efficacy is derived from the Albert Bandura's psychological research. The self-efficacy theory, later named social cognitive theory, highlights the effect of self-perception on one's ability to perform particular behaviors.[15] The theory suggests commitment to a goal relates to how a person perceives their ability. The greater the self-efficacy, the greater their commitment to achieve these goals.[15]

Bandura theorized that there are 4 major sources of self-efficacy. The first source of self-efficacy is through experiences overcoming obstacles. This is considered the strongest way to form self-efficacy.[15] The second source of self-efficacy is through modeling. Modeling is a social mirroring. It allows one to see others, similar to themselves, who are successfully performing the desired task or goal. The third source of self-efficacy is self-belief. This can be further supported by verbal encouragement from by an individual's social circle. The fourth source of self-efficacy is mastery

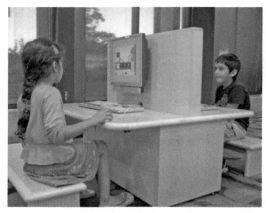

Fig. 4. The Indiana University School of Medicine (IU) created the Child Health Improvement through Computer Automation also known as the CHICA System. The program is a computerized decision-support system and an electronic medical record (EMR) for pediatric preventative. The CHICA system provides age-appropriate screening of patients in the waiting room via a tablet and then combining this information with electronic medical record data that generate patient-specific recommendations and reminders for the physician.[14] (San José Public Library. Children using computers. Flickr. Retrieved from: https://www.flickr.com/photos/sanjoselibrary/2839901913/.)

of an individual's physiologic state. An individual's negative emotions can lead to misinterpreting their physiologic states. For example, when a patient is anxious, they may be less confident that they can successfully meet a health care goal. People who believe they can manage their emotions are less likely to be less distressed by them.[15]

A high sense of self-efficacy leads to desired outcomes, such as improved health. It is recognized as a predictor of health behavior change and health maintenance.[15]

BEST PRACTICES AND STRATEGIES

a. Evidence Based Approaches and Strategies for Patient Education Within Preventative Health care

There are numerous evidence-based best practices and strategies for patient education within preventative health care including the promotion of health literacy, practicing a patient centered approach and utilizing technology (**Table 1**).[15]

Health Literacy

The health literacy of patients has been shown to significantly effect outcomes within preventative health care. When someone has lower health literacy, there has been an association with medication non-compliance, less utilization of preventative interventions like cancer screenings as well as a higher rate of hospitalizations.[20] Additionally, patients with limited health literacy have increased odds of being a smoker and are shown to be less likely to have had a mammogram.[22] Thus, patient education that promotes health literacy is an important tool in preventative medicine.

The United States Department of Health and Human Services defines personal health literacy as "the degree to which individuals have the ability to find, understand, and use information and services to inform health-related decisions and actions for themselves and others."[23] Health literacy includes a variety of skills including reading,

Table 1
Evidence-based approaches for preventative

Team-Based Care	Team-based approach is not a new approach for preventative care services. Recent studies have emphasized design, implementation, and evaluation of interprofessional health care teams. These teams may include specialist like endocrinologist and nurse educators with the goal of improving health outcomes and reducing costs.[16]
Patient-Oriented Care	Patient-oriented care increase patient compliance. In one study, patient-centered education increased adherence to treatment regimens of patients with coronary artery disease. Intervention groups received the standard patient education as well as 2 session of patient centered education. The control group only received the standard patient education. There was a significant difference between the 2 groups regarding treatment regimen adherence, which was measured in 3 dimensions including physical exercise, diet, and medication.[17]
Environmental Patient Education	According to one article, environmental patient education (ie, office-based videos, pamphlets, and posters) without individual staff or educator has not been well established in regard to increasing patient compliance. To maximize care, one should facilitate access to qualified medical educators and groups within the patient's community.[18]
Technology	Use of technology can improve communication of preventive recommendations. Incorporation of mobile apps has been proven to significantly increase medication adherence of preventative medication for cardiovascular disease (CVD). This is pivotal when adherence is reported to be only 57% in CVD, and when CVD attributes to about one-third of all deaths globally.[19]
Health Literacy	It has been found that health literacy is an independent predictor of participation in screenings for cervical, colorectal, and breast cancer.[20] One study found mammogram use was higher at 6 months in those whose intervention included an educational video, a coaching tool, recommendations given verbally and a written brochure compared to those whose intervention only included a written brochure and recommendations given verbally.[21]

Note: Brittany Stokes-Francis. Best Practice Strategies. 2024. Digital chart.
Adapted from Microsoft Corporation. Cloud Computing. 2023. Digital Commons image. Accessed December 1, 2023.

understanding, and analyzing information as well as comprehending instructions, charts, symbols, and diagrams. In addition, health literacy involves weighing risks and benefits and finally making choices and acting.[23]

Low health literacy regarding cancer screening may be due to decreased capacity to read and understand the material, difficulty comprehending the communications regarding risks, and ineffective approaches to prevention; thus, it is important that clinicians focus on this issue.[20] Providers determine the parameters of a health interaction, which in turn contributes to a patient's health literacy. Parameters include the physical setting, time spent with the patient, communication styles, modes of information, content, and decision-making concepts.[24] *The Agency for Health care Research*

Box 1
Best practices guidelines for (A) communication strategies supporting health literacy[25,38] and (B) additional strategies supporting health literacy[25]

A. Communication Strategies Supporting Health Literacy:[25,38]
- Use plain language and avoid medical jargon. Use words that the patient uses to describe their own health.
- Utilize visual aids like videos, models, diagrams, and pictures.
- Focus only on the information that the patient needs (3–5 key points).
- Listen carefully without interruption.
- Engage patients by encouraging questions.
- Ensure understanding through The Teach Me Back method: provider asks the patient or family member to tell them in their own words what they have been told during the medical encounter.
- Provide language interpretation.
- Simplify written communication: provide information in different languages and through using simple words.

B. Additional Strategies Supporting Health Literacy:[25]
- Create a welcoming, safe environment that is shame-free.
  - This pertains to every aspect of the patient encounter including phone calls, waiting rooms, examination rooms, and finance areas.
  - Examples: offering assistance with filling out forms, navigating patient portals.
- Decrease the digital divide.
  - Examples: Offer technical support, provide access to those who do not have personal devices, offer digital kiosks.
- Establish mechanisms to support patient's health management.
  - Examples: create action plans, provide medication guides, supply pill organizers.
- Provide training to staff at every level on the best practices for health literacy.
- Conduct Health Literacy Assessments to identify areas of weakness.

---

and Quality provides strategies for providers to improve health literacy, which are summarized in **Box 1**.[25]

Patient or Person-centered Care

Patient or person-centered approaches to patient education are beneficial in preventative health outcomes. Person-centered care is where "individuals' values and preferences are elicited and, once expressed, guide all aspects of their health care, supporting their realistic health and life goals. Person-centered care is achieved through a dynamic relationship among individuals, others who are important to them, and all relevant providers. This collaboration informs decision-making to the extent that the individual desires."[26] Evidence shows that better health outcomes during consultations are achieved using person-centered approaches to patient education. A person-centered educational approach differs from the traditional doctor centered educational approach, where the provider does the majority of the talking and uses professional status and persuasion as tools.[27] *See* **Box 2** for Patient-Centered Strategies for Patient Education within Preventative Medicine.

The Use of Technology and Patient Education

Digital health provides opportunities for patient education and supporting lifestyle changes. Information can be provided in the traditional forms like articles or as seen in digital health, through newer forms like multimedia including video, audio, and interactive videogames. Digital health encompasses a variety of technologies

---

Box 2
Best practices guidelines for patient-centered strategies for patient education within preventative medicine[27]

- Include lifestyle matters on the agenda of a medical visit. Allow the patient to take part in deciding if this is a discussion that they would like to proceed with.

- Engage in a discussion of risks and symptoms that is adjusted to the patient's context.

- Elicit the patient's views first. Providing information that is built on the patient's existing knowledge is more successful than providing general information. If the existing knowledge is incorrect, it can be modified at that time and built upon.

- Identify problems that the patient may encounter and discuss solutions together.

- Engage in discussion with the patient. Discussion can motivate and empower a patient to make lifestyle changes.

- Engage in shared decision making. Use the patient's solutions rather than the provider's solutions, as this can empower the patient, leading to increased commitment and success.

---

including wearable devices, mobile health, health information technology, telehealth and telemedicine (**Fig. 5**).[28] See **Box 3** for examples of technology as educational tools.

CHALLENGES AND CONSIDERATIONS
Existing Challenges for Preventative Medicine

- In the United States, public health agencies are under-funded in regard to prevention.
- Medical schools and residencies put more emphasis on teaching diagnosis and disease management, over prevention.
- Insurance companies historically have not paid well for prevention.[29]
- There is a lack of time spent with patients by providers, which serves as barrier for detecting lifestyle risk factors.[30]
- There is minimal training in patient-centered communication[27] as well as in health literacy.

Cultural, Diversity, and Ethical Considerations in Patient Education Within Preventative Medicine

In today's health care climate there remains a multitude of cultural and diversity considerations as well as ethical considerations.

As discussed earlier in this article, health literacy plays a major role in the effectiveness of patient education. Low health literacy is more likely seen in racial and ethnic minorities, in older adults and those with lower educational attainment.[31] In addition, disparities in screening prevalence may be contributed to lower income, and decreased access to schooling. In a study exploring health literacy as a barrier to cervical cancer screening in immigrant Latinas in New York, it was found that women with low health literacy were 16.7 times less likely to have ever had a pap smear. Currently, communication regarding screenings relies heavily on written communication in the form of brochures, test results, referrals, prescriptions. Barriers included educational materials being at an unsuitably high reading level, education materials not being available in a person's native language and that screening recommendations were multifaceted.[32] To help mitigate these disparities, cultural competence can have a significant effect on patient engagement. Promoting

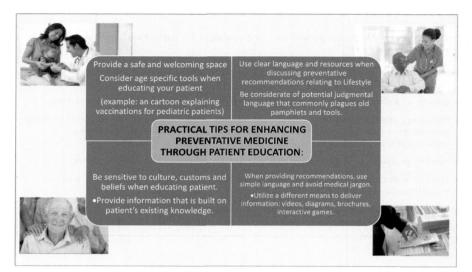

Fig. 5. Practical tips for enhancing preventative medicine through patient education.[25–28] Note: Brittany Stokes-Francis. Practical tips for enhancing preventative medicine through patient education. 2024. Digital chart. (*Adapted from* Microsoft Corporation. Cloud Computing. 2023. Digital Commons image. Accessed December 1, 2023.)

effective communication with diverse patient populations can be achieved through language assistance via interpreters, through cultural brokers who mediate between the practices of the patient's culture and traditional health beliefs, and through cultural competence training.[33]

Additional consideration should be given to digital health as utilizing electronic health may exacerbate health disparities in groups with limited technology skills and limited access to internet. Decreased access to internet has been reported in racial minorities, socioeconomically disadvantaged and older people.[30]

Regarding ethical considerations, there is a concern that patient education within preventative health care can increase unnecessary testing, which can be harmful to patients and increase costs. One study found that higher health literacy correlates to a higher rate of clinically unsupported cancer screenings for breast, cervical, and

---

Box 3
Technology as an educational tool example[28]

- *Text messages* can provide educational advice, support for changing lifestyle behaviors, and offer motivational reminders. Texts should keep in mind length, style of writing, literacy level, cultural and linguistic appropriateness.

- *Mobile Applications:* There were approximately 325,000 health related applications in 2017 with the majority focusing on healthy eating and physical activity. Applications can deliver education through providing insight into their lifestyle behaviors and through chances to develop new skills. Additionally, phones and tablets allow for visual education provided via games, videos, audio, and images.

- *Telemedicine:* Telemedicine increases access to education and support systems. It helps decrease barriers regarding access to care including those with decreased mobility.

prostate cancer. Inappropriate screenings for cancer in those with limited life expectancy is linked with overtreatment and diagnosis of indolent tumors, which can lead to adverse health outcomes with minimal survival benefit.[34]

FUTURE DIRECTIONS AND OPPORTUNITIES
Emerging Trends in Technology for Patient Education Within Preventative Medicine

Virtual and augmented reality

- This technology allows patients to implement new skills and behaviors through experiential learning.
- Example: One study utilized a tablet application in an augmented reality, which helped participants more accurately measure serving sizes compared to those who only received information.[35]

Artificial intelligence

- Machine learning can identify patterns in behavior data which can be utilized to predict the likelihood of future health outcomes.[28]
- Example: In one study, a novel artificial intelligence (AI) platform was used to measure and improve medication adherence in people who recently suffered an ischemic stroke. The application measured real-time medication adherence and the change in patient behavior. Ultimately, a 50% increase adherence was noted after using this AI platform.[35]

Recommendations

- There is a need for more awareness, resources, and funding to combat the barriers to patient education within preventative medicine.
- Training in patient-centered care and in health literacy is lacking throughout health care. It is important to encourage and support such training at every level within a health care organization.
- There is a need for research to focus more on clinical outcomes from medical adherence via technology, particularly mobile applications. Research should concentrate on the components of applications that make them successful when increasing medical adherence.[26]
- More emphasis should be placed on team-based care within health care systems to enhance patient education effectiveness.

SUMMARY

- Preventative medicine patient education is a valuable tool to better health outcomes, reduce costs, enhance patient experience while enhancing quality and safety.
- Evidence-based approaches to patient education within preventative medicine like team-based care and patient-centered care enhances patient education.
- There remain challenges and barriers within preventative medicine that continue to effect patient education which include: literacy, culture, language, and physiologic barriers.
- The HBM theory recognizes the value of avoiding illness utilizing the expectation that a behavior make aid in prevention or treatment.[10,11] It suggests that health care recommendations will have the largest patient population impact by targeting perceived barriers, benefits, self-efficacy, and threat.[11]

- The DOI theory encourages the application of high-technology media to provide evidence-based guidance.[28]
- The self-efficacy theory suggests commitment to a goal relates to how a person perceives their ability. The greater the self-efficacy, the greater their commitment to achieve these goals.[28]

CLINICS CARE POINTS

- Provide a safe and welcoming space.
- Suggest culturally sensitive and age specific tools when educating your patient.
- Use clear language and resources when discussing preventative recommendations relating to lifestyle.
- Be mindful of potential judgmental language that can plague old pamphlets and tools.
- Act as a team. Use clinic educators, specialist, and community resources to support preventative health recommendations.
- Provide information that is built on patient's existing knowledge.
- When providing recommendations, use simple language and avoid medical jargon.
- Utilize different means to deliver information: videos, diagrams, brochures, interactive games.

PRACTICAL RESOURCES

a. Self-efficacy, derived from Albert Bandura's psychological research is an important tool for preventative care education. He expands on his theory in the video below: Albert Bandura on Behavior Therapy, Self-Efficacy and Modeling Video.[36]
b. The Consumer Assessment of Health Care Providers and Systems (CAHPS) provides various surveys that offices, individuals, and organizations can use to identify areas in need of improvement regarding health literacy. Such surveys can be found on the CAHPS website. Please see references section for more information.[37]
c. The Office of Disease Prevention and Health Promotion website: https://health.gov/healthypeople/objectives-and-data/browse-objectives/preventive-care.

DISCLOSURE

The authors have nothing to disclose.

REFERENCES

1. Franklin's Philadelphia. Union Fire Company. ushistory.org. 2023. Available at: https://www.ushistory.org/franklin/philadelphia/fire.htm. [Accessed 8 December 2023].
2. Preventive medicine. Encyclopædia Britannica. Available at: https://www.britannica.com/science/preventive-medicine. [Accessed 20 November 2023].
3. Health care practices in ancient Greece: The Hippocratic ideal - PMC. PubMed Central (PMC. Available at: https://www.ncbi.nlm.nih.gov/pmc/articles/PMC4263393/. [Accessed 20 November 2023].
4. Preventive Medicine. Changing contexts and opportunities: academic medicine. LWW; 2000. Available at: https://journals.lww.com/academicmedicine/fulltext/2000/07001/preventive_medicine_2000__changing_contexts_and.4.aspx. [Accessed 20 November 2023].

5. Lynn B. Bates' guide to physical examination and history taking. Kindle Edition. Wolters Kluwer Health; 2022. p. 2.

6. Mass vaccination campaigns for polio eradication: an essential strategy for success - PubMed. Available at: https://pubmed.ncbi.nlm.nih.gov/16989271/. [Accessed 20 November 2023].

7. Schmidt H. Polio and covid-19: then and now from three polio survivors – Pennsylvania immunization coalition. Pennsylvania Immunization Coalition; 2022. Available at: https://www.immunizepa.org/polio-and-covid-19-then-and-now-from-three-polio-survivors/. [Accessed 17 September 2023].

8. Vaccine Hesitancy Course | Stanford Center for Continuing Medical Education | Stanford Medicine. Stanford Center for Continuing Medical Education. Available at: https://med.stanford.edu/cme/featured-programs/vaccine-hesitancy.html. [Accessed 15 October 2023].

9. Patient Education | AAFP. Home | AAFP. Available at: https://www.aafp.org/pubs/afp/issues/2000/1001/p1712.html. [Accessed 28 August 2023].

10. Glanz K, Rimer BK, Viswanath K. Health behavior67. John Wiley & Sons; 2015. p. 68.

11. The Health Belief Model as an explanatory framework in communication research: exploring parallel, serial, and moderated mediation - PubMed. Available at: https://pubmed.ncbi.nlm.nih.gov/25010519/. [Accessed 20 November 2023].

12. Dearing JW. Applying Diffusion of Innovation Theory to Intervention Development. Res Soc Work Pract 2009;(5):503–18. https://doi.org/10.1177/104973150933 35569.

13. Integration of diffusion of innovation theory into diabetes care - PubMed. Available at: https://pubmed.ncbi.nlm.nih.gov/27550077. [Accessed 20 November 2023].

14. The CHICA System | Children's Health Services Research Center | IU School of Medicine. Indiana University School of Medicine. Available at: https://medicine.iu.edu/pediatrics/specialties/health-services/child-health-informatics-research-development-lab/the-chica-system. [Accessed 15 November 2023].

15. Korpershoek C, van der Bijl J, Hafsteinsdóttir TB. Self-efficacy and its influence on recovery of patients with stroke: a systematic review. J Adv Nurs 2011;(9): 1876–94. https://doi.org/10.1111/j.1365-2648.2011.05659.x.

16. Enhancing primary care and preventive services through Interprofessional practice and education - PMC. PubMed Central (PMC). Available at: https://www.ncbi.nlm.nih.gov/pmc/articles/PMC7092466P. [Accessed 28 August 2023].

17. Saki M, Najmi S, Gholami M, et al. The effect of patient-centered education in adherence to the treatment regimen in patients with coronary artery disease. J Vasc Nurs 2021. https://doi.org/10.1016/j.jvn.2021.10.003.

18. Impact of environmental patient education on preventive medicine practices - PubMed. Available at: https://pubmed.ncbi.nlm.nih.gov/7699350/2. [Accessed 20 November 2023].

19. Al-Arkee S, Mason J, Lane DA, et al. Mobile Apps to Improve Medication Adherence in Cardiovascular Disease: Systematic Review and Meta-analysis. J Med Internet Res 2021;23(5). https://doi.org/10.2196/24190. N.PAG.

20. Baccolini V, Isonne C, Salerno C, et al. The association between adherence to cancer screening programs and health literacy: A systematic review and meta-analysis. Prev Med 2021. https://doi.org/10.1016/j.ypmed.2021.106927.

21. Berkman ND. Literacy and health outcomes. Agency for Healthcare Research and Quality; 2004.

22. Fernandez DM, Larson JL, Zikmund-Fisher BJ. Associations between health literacy and preventive health behaviors among older adults: findings from the health and retirement study. BMC Publ Health 2016;16:596. Published 2016 Jul 19.

23. Health Literacy. National Institutes of Health (NIH). 2021. Available at: https://www.nih.gov/institutes-nih/nih-office-director/office-communications-public-liaison/clear-communication/health-literacy. [Accessed 13 November 2023].

24. Paterick TE, Patel N, Tajik AJ, et al. Improving health outcomes through patient education and partnerships with patients. Proc (Bayl Univ Med Cent) 2017;30(1):112–3.

25. Strategies to Improve Organizational Health Literacy. PSNet 2023. Available at: https://psnet.ahrq.gov/primer/strategies-improve-organizational-health-literacy. [Accessed 13 November 2023].

26. Brummel SK, Butler D, Frieder M, et al. Person-Centered Care: A Definition and Essential Elements. J Am Geriatr Soc 2016;64(1):15–8. Available at: https://search-ebscohost-com.proxy-hs.researchport.umd.edu/login.aspx?direct=true&db=gnh&AN=EP112356951&site=eds-live. [Accessed 13 November 2023].

27. van Weel-Baumgarten E. Patient-centered information and interventions: tools for lifestyle change? Consequences for medical education. Family practice 2008;25(Suppl 1):i67–70.

28. Kuwabara A, Su S, Krauss J. Utilizing Digital Health Technologies for Patient Education in Lifestyle Medicine. Am J Lifestyle Med 2019;14(2):137–42.

29. Johnston RB. Promoting education is preventive medicine at its best. Pediatr Res 2020;87(2):185–7.

30. Carey M, Noble N, Mansfield E, et al. The Role of eHealth in Optimizing Preventive Care in the Primary Care Setting. J Med Internet Res 2015;17(5):e126.

31. Schillinger D, Bindman A, Wang F, et al. Functional health literacy and the quality of physician–patient communication among diabetes patients. Patient Educ Counsel 2004;52(3):315–23.

32. Garbers S, Chiasson MA. Inadequate functional health literacy in Spanish as a barrier to cervical cancer screening among immigrant Latinas in New York City. Prev Chronic Dis 2004;1(4):A07.

33. Cultural competence and patient safety. PSNet 2019. Available at: https://psnet.ahrq.gov/perspective/cultural-competence-and-patient-safety. [Accessed 13 November 2023].

34. Rutan MC, Sammon JD, Nguyen D-D, et al. The Relationship Between Health Literacy and Nonrecommended Cancer Screening. Am J Prev Med 2021;60(2):e69–72.

35. Labovitz DL, Shafner L, Reyes Gil M, et al. Using Artificial Intelligence to Reduce the Risk of Nonadherence in Patients on Anticoagulation Therapy. Stroke 2017;48(5):1416–9.

36. PsychotherapyNet. Albert Bandura on Behavior Therapy, Self-Efficacy and Modeling Video. 2014. Available at: https://www.youtube.com/watch?v=Km0RdJH_BP. [Accessed 20 November 2023].

37. Supplemental items for the CAHPS clinician & group adult survey 3.0: health literacy. Agency for Healthcare Research and Quality; 2017. Available at: https://www.ahrq.gov/cahps/surveys-guidance/item-sets/cg/suppl-healthlit-items-cg-survey30-adult.html. [Accessed 13 November 2023].

38. Teach-Back Intervention. Patient and family engagement in primary care. Agency for Healthcare Research and Quality; 2017. Available at: https://www.ahrq.gov/patient-safety/reports/engage/interventions/teachback.html. [Accessed 13 November 2023].

Patient Education and Special Populations: Part 1

Victoria Trott, MMS, PA-C, AQH[a],*, Mary Holthaus, MSPAS, PA-C[b,1]

KEYWORDS

- Developmentally disabled • Intellectually disabled • Geriatric • Patient education
- Special populations • Health literacy • Shared decision-making

KEY POINTS

- In this article, the authors discuss patient education with the focus inadvertently centering around or emphasizing the patient's health concerns without inclusion of the patient's values.
- When considering patients with intellectually and developmentally disabled (IDD) or those in the aging population, it is important to implement strategies and utilize tools that focus on quality of life for the patient, caregivers, and the support network. In health care, use of varied approaches permits flexibility and adaptation to better meet the individualized nature of the patient's needs.
- In this article, topics addressed for the patients of the IDD and geriatric populations include the following: background, best practices and strategies, challenges, and future considerations.
- The goal of the article is to provide insight into these populations regarding evidence-based strategies that can be implemented into everyday practice and improve patient outcomes.
- Ultimately, IDD and aging populations are vulnerable, and identifying ways to improve health literacy and subsequently health outcomes is essential to mitigate potential and inadvertent harm.

INTRODUCTION

Patient education during clinical interactions helps to improve health behaviors and clinical outcomes.[1] When discussing patient education, the focus may inadvertently center around or emphasize the patient's health concerns without inclusion of the patient's values. Patients benefit when health care providers (HCPs) take into account their health literacy. Low health literacy negatively impacts patient's physical and cognitive wellness.[2] Therefore, HCPs may need to consider an individualized approach to

[a] University of Maryland, Baltimore, USA; [b] Virginia Commonwealth University Medical Center
[1] Present address: 9105 Stony Point Drive, Richmond, VA 23235.
* Correspondent author. 520 West Fayette Street, Suite 100, Baltimore, MD 21201.
E-mail address: vtrott@umaryland.edu

Physician Assist Clin 9 (2024) 567–576
https://doi.org/10.1016/j.cpha.2024.05.008
2405-7991/24/Published by Elsevier Inc.

patient education based on the subpopulation. When considering patients with IDD or those in the aging population, it is important to implement strategies and utilize tools that focus on quality of life for the patient, caregivers, and the support network. In health care, use of varied approaches permits flexibility and adaptation to better meet the individualized nature of the patient's needs.

Throughout the remainder of the article, topics addressed for the patients of the IDD and geriatric populations include the following: background, best practices and strategies, challenges, and future considerations. The goal of the article is to provide insight into these populations regarding evidence-based strategies that can be implemented into everyday practice and improve patient outcomes. Ultimately, IDD and aging populations are vulnerable, and identifying ways to improve health literacy and subsequently health outcomes is essential to mitigate potential and inadvertent harm.

BACKGROUND AND CONTEXT

Historically, HCPs were often viewed as the authority figure in the patient–provider relationship. The HCPs would determine the appropriate history, physical examination, and treatment plan without the patient's input. Until the 1960s, the concept of active patient participation in their care was less prevalent.[3] Over the next 2 decades, a greater emphasis was placed on patient education as a component of treatment planning. In the mid of the growing movement surrounding more active patient involvement, understanding health literacy also became important in the 1970s. Health literacy is an individual's ability to interpret and utilize health information,[2,4] for example, following dietary recommendations for limiting sodium intake in congestive heart failure patients. Health literacy is influenced by social determinants of health (eg, education, support, financial) and can also change over the course of a person's life.[2,4] In the 1980s, there were patient advocacy groups, a growing understanding of health literacy and routinely implementing patient education during appointments.[3,5] Today, patient education has expanded through policy, research, community outreach, and educating health professionals.[3]

Although the health care landscape involving patients' self-awareness of their health has improved, there remains a need for optimizing how patient education is conveyed and understood by different subpopulations. Low health literacy is associated with lower self-reported physical and cognitive functioning.[6] For example, a 70 year old patient with mild cognitive impairment who is living alone and recently underwent surgery is at risk of complications if without a clear strategy for adapted patient education for their individualized care needs.

THEORETIC FOUNDATIONS
Intellectually and Developmentally Disabled and Geriatric Populations

There is overlap within IDD and older adult subpopulations when recognizing the impact of health literacy on an HCP's approach to patient care and education. Utilizing health literacy models may support patient adherence and improve health outcomes in these subpopulations.

One model to consider is Nutbeam's tripartite model (**Table 1**), which provides a way to monitor the development of health literacy.[9] This model depicts health literacy as an outcome of health education utilizing 3 distinct dimensions.[4] One dimension (eg, critical health literacy) expands health literacy beyond the individual to include the empowerment of a community.[7] Providers referencing this model as a guide may have an understanding of the individual and social impacts on the patient's health literacy, care, and education.

Table 1
Nutbeam's tripartite model[4,7,8]

Dimension	Definition	Example
Functional Health Literacy	Evaluating the ability of reading, writing, and numeracy skills to interpret the health information provided	Barrier to communication: Providing patient instructions in their native language
Interactive Health Literacy	An individual's ability to understand the information and apply to self-care and self-management	Demonstration: Patient shows proper use of inhaler for asthma in the clinical setting
Critical Health Literacy	Empowers an individual and community to work together in both a social and political way in attempts to improve health inequalities	Advocacy: Encouraging participation in a community 5K walk/run to raise awareness for Parkinson's disease

An additional model of benefit for the aforementioned subpopulations was developed by Sørensen and colleagues,[7] whereby health literacy, its impact on patient care and outcomes involve an integrative approach. This model demonstrates the link between the health literacy of the patient, factors impacting the health literacy of the patient, and how a provider may present information in a way that the patient may understand and apply. Providers can utilize the model as a guide when identifying health literacy concerns within patients of the IDD and aging populations and how to address these concerns. Low health literacy can be associated with cognitive changes in the patient, living alone or with another elderly spouse, language barriers, education, social systems, and family and peer or media influences.[2,7] Identifying these barriers during early clinical interactions allows for modifications to patient education, for example, limiting the number of recommendations and encouraging simple tasks to complete.[7] With each subsequent appointment, the provider builds upon that foundation. If there are cognitive challenges, both the patient and their support system should be included in the conversation in a manner that both can understand and implement at home. Improving health literacy among patients could lead to improvement in one's personal life and societal change.[7]

BEST PRACTICES AND STRATEGIES
Intellectually and Developmentally Disabled Population

Standard of care for HCPs providing high-quality patient care involves evidence-based medicine. When considering how to best approach the patient, family/caregiver/surrogate decision-maker, and the HCP may integrate these evidence-based strategies, this includes provider–patient communication, care plan structure, and patient support.[10] For example, the HCP should remain focused, communicate in a direct way, and utilize pictures, objects, technology, and videos. Structuring a plan using a limited number of tasks and allowing for adaptations as needed can improve adherence. Patient support from HCPs and caregivers also improves outcomes, giving a sense of hope and encouragement to the patient.[10] Actively listening to their needs, creating a plan that is obtainable and being supportive may lead to a better patient–provider relationship and health outcomes. HCPs can refer to the IDD Toolkit created in collaboration with the Vanderbilt Kennedy Center for Research on Human Development, the University of Tennessee Boling Center for Developmental Disabilities, and the Tennessee Department of

Intellectual and Developmental Disabilities. The IDD Toolkit provides patient education guidance to HCPs when caring for patients with IDD and resources for patients and their families or caregivers.[11]

Another consideration involves the family, caregivers, or surrogate decision-makers ability to improve their own support skills. One evidence-based practice that can assist is the La Trobe Support for Decision-making Practice Framework. In this framework, there are steps and strategies that focus on the preferences of the patient and guide those that are making decisions. Studies have shown that exploring outside viewpoints assists caregivers when they are making health care decisions.[12] As is displayed in **Table 2**, this framework acts as a checklist that considers the patient, the decision, and the patient's preference for the decision, considering challenges and refining the decision, identifying the need for a formal process, and determining and then implementing the decision.[12,13] Although the framework may seem geared toward the patient's direct support system, it can also guide HCPs. Therefore, having knowledge of the framework in the clinical setting and recommending it as a resource could be invaluable.

HCPs may learn these strategies and apply them into everyday practice. The La Trobe Support for Decision-making Practice Framework steps are applied to patient scenario examples in the following.

Geriatric Population

HCPs are familiar with a shared decision-making or patient-centered care approach to creating medical treatment plans. In geriatric populations, there often is a need for a triadic model to include the provider, patient, and caregiver. This requires a balance between patient and caregiver preferences when choosing treatments.[14] Patients may begin the discussion of advanced care planning with family, caregivers, or surrogate decision-makers prior to the onset of significant physical or cognitive decline. Advanced care planning with patients of the aging population supports inclusivity of their wishes; health preferences are established and continue to be considered as caregivers' medical decision-making responsibility increases.[3,15] Another tool that can be used in offices, hospital units, and emergency rooms is the comprehensive geriatric assessment (CGA). The CGA helps HCPs identify patient medical and

Table 2 La Trobe support for decision-making practice framework[12,13]	
Framework Steps	**Patient Scenario Example**
Patient	Identifying the patient and caregiver
Decision	Diagnosing the patient with hypertension and discussing initiation of an antihypertensive medication with the patient and caregiver
Patient's Preference	The patient/caregiver prefers once-a-day dosing of medication
Challenges and Refining the Decision	Reviewing antihypertensive medications with an option of once-a-day dose
Identifying the need for a Formal Process	Ensure patient and caregiver preferences align and do not result in harm to the patient or others
Determining the Decision	Choosing an appropriate antihypertensive medication
Implementing the Decision	Prescribing medication with detailed administration instructions and providing resources to patients and caregivers

functional needs and then create appropriate care plans. Components of the CGA are incorporated into the Medicare Annual Wellness Exam that allows for personalized treatment plans with the primary care team. When the CGA is used in acute care evaluations in the hospital and emergency departments, it is associated with positive outcomes based on observational studies. For example, acute care units reported reductions in length of stay, costs, incidence of delirium, mortality, and readmissions. In emergency departments, utilizing CGA has been linked to reduced admissions to intensive care unit, increased referrals for palliative care, and increased patient satisfaction.[16]

Two areas of focus for improving geriatric patient–provider communication involve training the HCP teams and caregivers through programs or workshops. A cohort observational study identified patient and caregiver concerns regarding HCP communication, which included conveying all information required for the shared decision-making process, establishing and managing expectations, and discussing care plans with compassion and empathy.[17] The Comskil Laboratory at Memorial Sloan Kettering Cancer Center created the Geriatric Shared Decision Making module to optimize communication skills of HCPs with patients.[14] Enhanced informal caregiver training can improve caregiver self-efficacy regarding symptom and stress management.[18] The Care Talks program created by Smith and colleagues[19] aimed to hold workshops to improve caregiver confidence regarding communication with HCPs. The 3 components for shared decision-making involve "declaring the agenda," "inviting the agenda," and "checking preference." Creating a structure for patient visits allows the patient and caregiver to know what to expect when attending appointments. Inviting the agenda sets aside time for the patient and caregivers to ask and discuss topics regarding their health and care plan. The Care Talks program encouraged caregivers to compose their questions and talking points prior to visits so they can be addressed appropriately. Checking preferences will confirm the treatment goals are matching the patient's values.[14] Incorporating reflective listening ensures the patient and caregiver understands the treatment plan and goals to reduce misunderstandings.

Another step for clarifying treatment goals includes providing printout summaries that highlight important takeaways from the visit. This allows patients and caregivers to review information that was discussed and document sustainable treatment plans or patient goals such as lifestyle modifications.[2,17] Special considerations should be made when creating visit summaries for patients with hearing, visual, or cognitive impairments or language differences. Information provided should have clear, concise language based on the patient's health literacy status. Patients with hearing impairments would benefit from printed summaries to reference and review when needed. For patients with visual impairment such as macular degeneration, print can be enlarged and a copy of the visit summary can be provided to designated caregivers if necessary. For those with cognitive impairments, such as dementia, the language on the printed visit summaries is adapted to the patients' and the caregivers' health literacy. Caregiver involvement in education and care planning has shown positive outcomes in patients with cognitive impairment.[20]

Based on evidence-based practices, **Table 3** summarizes key components when creating a patient-centered care plan through shared decision-making.

CHALLENGES AND CONSIDERATIONS
Intellectually and Developmentally Disabled and Geriatric Populations

There are several challenges that can impact health outcomes in IDD and aging populations. These challenges involve health care resources, patients' attitudes, and

Table 3
Navigating patient-centered care plan[10,14,21]

Components	Clinical Practices
Communication	1. Be sure to have patient's attention 2. Be clear and to the point 3. Consider using gestures 4. Limit outside stimuli, that is, too much noise
Plan and Patient Education	1. Consider use of visual aids 2. Create a plan appropriate for patient's level of understanding 3. Limit the number of items to improve practice time 4. Include the patient's values into the plan
Support	1. Work closely with parents, caregivers, and/or surrogate decision-makers 2. Recommend working in groups and provide resources 3. Be supportive and provide encouragement

patients' support systems. Research has shown that patients with IDD experience higher rates of disease, chronic illnesses, and language deficits, which require a significant level of support from caregivers.[4,22] Currently, evidence-based practice is limited in the IDD populations and has been generalized from the mental health field even if not applicable which creates challenges for the patient, family, and HCPs.[23] Successful HCPs are mindful to include both the patient and caregiver in the conversation. They also must be aware that low health literacy, personal health and attitudes, and lack of resources are challenges seen in the support network.[24] HCPs may recognize that the support network may also have barriers, which limits their abilities to incorporate the education provided into the patient's daily routine and then create treatment plans accordingly.

There are further challenges with implementation of evidence-based practice among health care providers due to lack of knowledge and preconceived beliefs or opinions, as well as communication barriers.[25] Additional training for HCPs may be required to improve competency when administering health screening tools such as the IDD Toolkit or the CGA.[2,11,16] Many offices and acute care units experience time restraints and lack the dedicated time required for counseling patients and caregivers during visits or interactions to allow for reflective listening. Geriatric patients may have decreased ability to understand the patient education provided due to cognitive, visual, or hearing impairment resulting in misunderstanding.[2,14] HCPs may invite family members or caregivers into the discussion and treatment plan sooner to reduce risk for unclear instructions.[14] Some regions may lack the community support resources for caregiver training in IDD and geriatric populations. Increasing awareness of the functional health and social benefits for providing facility and community resources could allow for allocation of funding for these programs to improve health literacy and patient education.

In both IDD and aging populations, there are ethical considerations that may impact the interaction between a patient and the provider. Ethical considerations include determining competency and decision-making capacity of the patient and surrogate decision-making.[26,27] If the patient is unable to make a decision, understand the consequences of the decision, and reason with prior values, there is a concern that the patient lacks capacity. Concern for decision-making capacity can be identified in IDD and older adult populations with cognitive impairment. Patients with IDD or cognitive impairment may be agreeable to the plan despite lack of understanding.[26] If capacity is brought into question, HCPs may consult other health care professionals, such as psychiatrists and social workers.[27] When these patients rely on their care-givers, surrogate decision-making ethics must be assessed. Concerns may arise if surrogate decision-makers are not acting in the best interest of the patient. In these situations, the HCP may have had prior knowledge of the patient's values and will need to address changes in the patient preferences with the surrogate decision-maker. If there is not a designated surrogate decision-maker, the HCP may be respon-sible for determining who would be the best candidate for this role. Studies have shown that the patient's values and treatment decisions are not always known by the surrogate decision-makers, and in turn, health-related decisions are based on the surrogate decision-maker's values.[27] Although there are other ethical dilemmas that will likely present themselves in practice, it is important to utilize the array of re-sources (ie, social work, case manager, lawyers) that may be available to assist in these situations and ultimately will provide the best course for the patient.

Cultural and diversity can impact a patient's health literacy. The model presented by Sørensen, and colleagues[7] refers to the primary definition of health literacy and shows the impact of distal factors, such as environmental and societal determinants (eg, culture, language), as well as proximal factors, such as personal and situational deter-minants (eg, education, race). Among older adults, education has been shown to correlate with health literacy.[2] Clinical trials are scarce for IDD and aging populations, and of those studies there is minimal diversity.[2,24] Research inclusion/exclusion criteria often omit these subpopulations, making it difficult to accurately identify the impact of patient education, health literacy, and health outcomes.[6,24] With limited research avail-able to HCPs, it makes educating these subpopulations more challenging.

FUTURE DIRECTIONS AND OPPORTUNITIES
Intellectually and Developmentally Disabled and Geriatric Populations

Health care is rapidly advancing each year, though improvements are ever ongoing. An emerging area involves the use of artificial intelligence (AI) and extended reality (XR).[28,29] HCPs may use AI tools to analyze a patient's facial expressions or record their voice to obtain further medical data and provide insight on when assessing phar-macologic or behavioral therapies.[28] Through video analysis with AI, Kobayashi and colleagues[30] revealed multimodal comprehensive communication skills training increased time spent by physicians performing single and multimodal communication skills. AI technology can also be used for identifying and diagnosing various conditions in geriatric patients. These patients may start necessary treatments sooner than tradi-tional diagnostic assessments. Research is in-progress to assess mental health research and care, assessment of early signs of cognitive impairment, and identifying risk factors for frailty syndrome.[8,31] AI may provide options, such as games, for cogni-tive training, which may improve cognition and behavior.[28] Research has shown that individuals with mild-to-moderate IDD can benefit from XR particularly when consid-ering practical skills, such as activities of daily living, as well as cognitive and physical skills.[29] Ultimately, integration and utilization of multimodal AI and XR programs for these subpopulations may assist HCPs in diagnosis, formulating a treatment plan, and improving patient adherence and health outcomes.

Future research may consider adaptations to the study design and exclusion criteria to include the IDD and older adult populations for studies assessing effective patient education. Additionally, research could also focus on the perspective of both the IDD and geriatric subpopulations and caregivers.[20,32] Caregiver education is a key compo-nent to comprehensive patient education in these subpopulations.[20] Primary outcome goals in research could reflect what patients and caregivers deem important or beneficial regarding treatments. Unless feedback is given to HCPs, health disparities remain.

SUMMARY

Ultimately, patient empowerment is an integral component of an HCP's role, which encourages patients to actively participate in their own medical care through appropriate and individualized patient education. To provide quality, patient-centered care to the IDD and geriatric populations, HCPs must develop a strategy for care planning and patient education that includes both patients and caregivers. Utilizing resources such as the IDD Toolkit or the CGA can guide HCPs to customize the patient's education and plan to best address the patient's needs.

CLINICS CARE POINTS

- Utilization of the IDD Toolkit can provide patient education guidance to HCPs and resources for IDD patients and their families or caregivers.
- The CGA can assist HCPs identify patient medical and functional needs and create appropriate care plans.
- Consider involving and actively engaging the patient, family and caregivers in the shared-decision making process.
- Additional training for HCPs may be required to improve competency when administering health screenings tools, such as IDD Toolkit or the CGA.

DISCLOSURE

The authors have no conflicts to disclose.

REFERENCES

1. Eckman MH, Wise R, Leonard AC, et al. Impact of health literacy on outcomes and effectiveness of an educational intervention in patients with chronic diseases. Patient Education and Counseling 2012;87(2):143–51.
2. Kim MY, Oh S. Nurses' perspectives on health education and health literacy of older patients. Int J Environ Res Public Health 2020;17(18):6455.
3. Hoving C, Visser A, Mullen PD, et al. A history of patient education by health professionals in Europe and North America: from authority to shared decision making education. Patient education and counseling 2010;78(3):275–81.
4. Geukes C, Bröder J, Latteck ÄD. Health literacy and people with intellectual disabilities: what we know, what we do not know, and what we need: a theoretical discourse. Int J Environ Res Public Health 2019;16(3):463.
5. Wittink H, Oosterhaven J. Patient education and health literacy. Musculoskeletal Science and Practice 2018;38(1):120–7.
6. Chesser AK, Keene Woods N, Smothers K, et al. Health literacy and older adults: a systematic review. Gerontol Geriatr Med 2016;2. 2333721416630492.
7. Sørensen K, Van den Broucke S, Fullam J, et al, (HLS-EU) Consortium Health Literacy Project European. Health literacy and public health: a systematic review and integration of definitions and models. BMC Public Health 2012;12:80.

8. Velazquez-Diaz D, Arco JE, Ortiz A, et al. Use of artificial intelligence in the identification and diagnosis of frailty syndrome in older adults: scoping review. J Med Internet Res 2023;25:e47346.

9. Velardo S. The nuances of health literacy, nutrition literacy, and food literacy. J Nutr Educ Behav 2015-Aug;47(4):385–9.e1.

10. Evidence-based Practices for IDD | NC Complex Mental Health and Intellectual Developmental Disabilities Resources. complexmhidd-nc.org. Available at: https://complexmhidd-nc.org/physical-behavioral-healthcare.

11. Muccilli K. Health care for adults with intellectual and developmental disabilities: toolkit for primary care providers. Available at: https://iddtoolkit.vkcsites.org/. [Accessed 13 November 2023].

12. Bigby C, Douglas J, Smith E, et al. I used to call him a non-decision-maker - I never do that anymore": parental reflections about training to support decision-making of their adult offspring with intellectual disabilities. Disabil Rehabil 2022;44(21):6356–64.

13. Douglas J, Bigby C. Development of an evidence-based practice framework to guide decision making support for people with cognitive impairment due to acquired brain injury or intellectual disability. Disabil Rehabil 2020;42(3):434–41.

14. Shen MJ, Manna R, Banerjee SC, et al. Incorporating shared decision making into communication with older adults with cancer and their caregivers: development and evaluation of a geriatric shared decision-making communication skills training module. Patient Educ Couns 2020;103(11):2328–34.

15. Lum HD, Sudore RL, Bekelman DB. Advance care planning in the elderly. Medical Clinics of North America 2015;99(2):391–403.

16. Parker SG, McLeod A, McCue P, et al. New horizons in comprehensive geriatric assessment. Age Ageing 2017;46(5):713–21.

17. Huang SC-C, Morgan A, Peck V, et al. Improving communications with patients and families in geriatric care. The how, when, and what. Journal of Patient Experience 2021;8. https://doi.org/10.1177/23743735211034047.

18. Hendrix CC, Bailey DE Jr, Steinhauser KE, et al. Effects of enhanced caregiver training program on cancer caregiver's self-efficacy, preparedness, and psychological well-being. Support Care Cancer 2016;24(1):327–36.

19. Smith PD, Martin B, Chewning B, et al. Improving health care communication for caregivers: a pilot study. Gerontol Geriatr Educ 2018-Dec;39(4):433–44.

20. Garcia-Ptacek S, Dahlrup B, Edlund AK, Wijk H, et al. The caregiving phenomenon and caregiver participation in dementia. Scand J Caring Sci 2019;33(2):255–65.

21. Kauffman JM, Hung LY. Special education for intellectual disability: current trends and perspectives. Current Opinion in Psychiatry 2009;22(5):452–6.

22. Krahn GL, Hammond L, Turner A. A cascade of disparities: Health and health care access for people with intellectual disabilities. Mental Retardation and Developmental Disabilities Research Reviews 2006;12(1):70–82.

23. Man J, Kangas M. Best practice principles when working with individuals with intellectual disability and comorbid mental health concerns. Qual Health Res 2020;30(4):560–71.

24. Turnbull H, Dark L, Carnemolla P, Skinner I, Hemsley B. A systematic review of the health literacy of adults with lifelong communication disability: looking beyond accessing and understanding information. Patient Educ Couns 2023;106:151–62.

25. Lennox NG, Kerr MP. Primary health care and people with an intellectual disability: the evidence base. J Intellect Disabil Res 1997;41(Pt 5):365–72.

26. Carlson L. Research ethics and intellectual disability: broadening the debates. Yale J Biol Med 2013;86(3):303–14.
27. Mueller PS, Hook CC, Fleming KC. Ethical issues in geriatrics: a guide for clinicians. Mayo Clin Proc 2004;79(4):554–62.
28. Krysta K, Romańczyk M, Diefenbacher A, et al. Telemedicine treatment and care for patients with intellectual disability. Int J Environ Res Public Health 2021;18(4): 1746.
29. Maran PL, Daniëls R, Slegers K. The use of extensive reality (XR) for people with moderate to severe intellectual disabilities (ID): a scoping review. Technology and Disability 2022;1–15.
30. Kobayashi M, Katayama M, Hayashi T, et al. Effect of multimodal comprehensive communication skills training with video analysis by artificial intelligence for physicians on acute geriatric care: a mixed-methods study. BMJ Open 2023;13(3): e065477.
31. Renn BN, Schurr M, Zaslavsky O, Pratap A. Artificial intelligence: an interprofessional perspective on implications for geriatric mental health research and care. Front Psychiatry 2021;12:734909.
32. Feldman MA, Aunos M. Recent trends and future directions in research regarding parents with intellectual and developmental disabilities. Current Developmental Disorders Reports 2020;7(3):173–81.

Patient Education and Special Populations: Part 2

ToriAnne M. Yetter, DMS, PA-C, PMH-C, CLSP

KEYWORDS

- Perinatal • Mental health • Primary care • Minority populations • Care setting
- Postpartum outcomes

KEY POINTS

- Perinatal mental health is not adequately screened.
- Perinatal mental health education is limited, especially for minority populations.
- Optimizing perinatal mental health will lead to improved postpartum outcomes for parent and baby.
- Perinatal mental health can be safely addressed in a primary care setting by physicians and advanced practice clinicians with the appropriate threshold for referral.

INTRODUCTION

Proper mental health and wellness remain in the limelight of clinicians' attention as it is increasingly recognized as a catalyst for maintaining physical health. Unfortunately, psychiatric services are not as readily available as one's primary care provider.[1] Despite primary care clinicians acting as the first line of management, there has been limited research into how primary care providers can adequately assess and treat perinatal mental health disorders.[2] In treating mental health in the perinatal context, it is vital to educate the patient on the risks and benefits of medication treatment while being cautious not to coerce patients into a decision that is not comfortable for them. For the birthing parent, medication treatment can be fraught with guilt and should be pursued with the highest level of insight and education from the provider. Further compounding barriers to receiving education, patients may avoid the clinic secondary to stigmatization.[3] In conjunction with medication education, health care providers may consider the value of nonpharmacological options such as therapy, support groups, mind–body exercises, and alternative therapies such as aromatherapy.[4]

BACKGROUND

Becoming a parent involves a monumental transition known as matrescence.[5] Society tends to highlight the positive aspects of parenthood while downplaying the trials and

620 West Lexington Street, Baltimore, MD 21201, USA
E-mail address: davies.torianne@gmail.com

Physician Assist Clin 9 (2024) 577–588
https://doi.org/10.1016/j.cpha.2024.05.009
2405-7991/24/© 2024 Elsevier Inc. All rights are reserved, including those for text and data mining, AI training, and similar technologies.

tribulations that both the pregnant parent and the nonpregnant parent experience.[6] While more commonly thought of in the female population, perinatal mood and anxiety disorders (PMADs) can also affect male and other nonbinary parents and parents-to-be.[7,8] The lack of perinatal mental health equity among marginalized populations, specifically the lesbian, gay, bisexual, transgender, and queer+ community, highlights an even more significant deficit.[7,8]

There is research to suggest that 1 in 7 new parents will develop a PMAD, with the second leading cause of death in the first-year postpartum being suicide.[9,10] According to the Centers for Disease Control and Prevention data collected from the Pregnancy Risk Assessment and Monitoring System, it has been identified that between 20% and 30% of pregnant persons are not asked about their mental health during pregnancy and at the 6 week follow-up.[11] To educate patients about perinatal mental health, recognition is crucial.

Perinatal is defined as the time from conception to 1 year postpartum, with loose definitions for the makeup of the antepartum population.[12] Perinatal mental health has historically been thought of in terms of postpartum depression.[12] While that is one specific example of PMADs, these conditions span a much more vast territory of wellness. The state of preconception mental health has much to do with intrapartum and postpartum mental states and may be one of the strongest predictors of morbidity.[13]

Advanced practice clinicians (APCs) have the unique opportunity to work toward improving mental health with a broad and thorough education base across the primary care realm. As the lens of mental health awareness is just beginning to clear, the attention to the perinatal population has not yet come into focus. The clinician should have trauma-informed answers to the hard questions from our birthing and non-birthing patients who are beginning the journey into parenthood.

This article identifies and differentiates between different PMADs, reflects on options for management and patient education, and prompts the clinician to consider when and who to refer to for care escalation. For this article, the focus will be directed toward education for the most common perinatal mood disorders, with recognition of other common but deserving peripartum mental illnesses for thoroughness.

DISCUSSION
Patient Identification

By asking well-informed questions and conscientiously evaluating the patient's demeanor, clinicians in primary care can identify teaching points that can significantly improve the mental health of the perinatal population. Patients in the postpartum may not understand how to navigate the fragmented health care system, and when interacting with primary care providers, mental health is not addressed.[14] Pediatric, family medicine, and obstetric clinicians should be aware of risk factors for poor perinatal mental health, identifying populations that may require more probing. These include patients who have experienced a mental health condition in the past, such as anxiety or depression.[15] External to historical mental health illness and genetic predispositions, patients in minority populations experience the most risk for progressive mental health; specifically black women.[16] Patients lacking social support, financial constraints, and those with neurodivergence are also at increased risk of PMADs.[17,18] A history of intimate partner violence should prompt the clinician to think critically about that patient's risks for mental health disorders.[19]

Traditionally, primary care providers have utilized forms such as the PHQ-9 and GAD-7 to screen for depression and anxiety, respectively.[20] While these are great tools to use along the continuum of care for the perinatal population, other tools may provide more specific insight into the wellness of the parenting and pre-parenting patient. These include the 10 question Edinburgh Postnatal Depression Scale (EPDS) and the abbreviated 3 question EPDS.[21] Other helpful tools to consider include using mobile applications such as the Massachusetts General Hospital Perinatal Depression Scale application that can be downloaded and assessed by the patient at home or in the office.[22]

Differentiating Perinatal Mood and Anxiety Disorders and Symptom Validation

It is essential to differentiate between different expressions of PMADs both in the intrapartum and postpartum stages of the parenting population. Health care professional training has been identified as a barrier to implementing perinatal mental health education.[23] Intrapartum phenotypes of mood disorders in pregnant and postpartum patients can present with more variability.[24] If providers have a greater understanding of the nuances across different PMADs, they can provide the patient with individualized education and support.[25]

Postpartum depression

Postpartum depression must be contrasted with its more short-lived counterpart, baby blues, which is limited to 14 days duration and not considered to be a precursor to developing a PMAD.[26] The baby blues involve tearfulness, waxing, and waning moods that can be largely attributed to the sudden hormonal shift upon delivery of the placenta.[26] In contrast, postpartum depression meets the clinical criteria of depression in that there is low mood for most days of at least 2 weeks' duration as well as marked and diminished interest in activities previously enjoyed.[9] Postpartum depression can also involve feelings of worthlessness as a parent, inability to cope with parenting, and a sense of being trapped.[27] Many parents can become unglued during what is colloquially called the "witching hour."[27] A key hallmark of postpartum depression is the ability to sleep. Clinicians may find the following question fruitful: "if given a clean, cozy bed for 8 hours, would you be able to sleep?"[27] If the answer is no, there is a high likelihood that the patient is suffering from some degree of postpartum depression, as low-quality sleep causes over a 3 fold increase in developing postpartum depression.[28]

Postpartum anxiety

Related and often hand in hand with postpartum depression, postpartum anxiety is quite debilitating to the parenting population. However, postpartum anxiety symptoms usually present with a predominance of fear.[27] Fear about the baby, fear about one's mental and physical health, and fear of losing control.[27] These worries can be related to the baby's birthing process or entirely unrelated to parenthood.[27] Due to persistent worry, patients often report feeling keyed up, on edge, and tense, lending to irritability and a negative reactivity pattern.[27]

Obsessive-compulsive disorder

Once considered a type of anxiety disorder, obsessive-compulsive disorder is a compilation of symptoms and signs related to neuroticism, an independent risk factor for PMADs.[29] Postpartum obsessive-compulsive disorder includes both obsessions that are distressing and compulsions to alleviate that distress; these intrusive thoughts often surround concerns of harm to the baby or self, such as a knife dropping on the baby or falling down the stairs with the baby.[27] Parents may also find themselves preoccupied with diaper counts or engaging in excessive hand-washing rituals to avoid the spread of germs.[27] When thoughts surrounding violence or harm to the baby become sticky, the parent will often feel fearful that these things could genuinely happen.[27] There is a cognitive dissonance between the thoughts and the values and desires of the parent. This can lead to shame and a lack of reporting these thoughts to a provider. It is essential to ask patients about these thoughts and validate them as unrelated to their parenting ability.

Postpartum psychosis

It is crucial to differentiate intrusive thoughts from a state of postpartum psychosis, in which the parent is unable to separate the scary thoughts as discordant. Postpartum psychosis is a rare occurrence but a true medical emergency in which the baby and potentially the parent are at risk for harm secondary to detachment from reality.[27] Both delusions and hallucinations may occur.[27] There is no cognitive dissonance in the setting of postpartum psychosis; the thoughts of harm can feel necessary and may or may not be feared.[27]

Posttraumatic stress disorder

Posttraumatic stress disorder in the peripartum patient appears similar to the non-peripartum patient in that one may experience flashbacks to the trauma, reliving the event, hypervigilance, and increased arousal.[30] Specifically, it is important to ask the postpartum patient about any birth trauma they may have experienced, as this is a common but often overlooked form of trauma for many birthing parents.[31] Many birthing parents are discharged from the hospital in a state of shock and distress, taking with them stories that deserve to be unpacked in the appropriate setting.[31]

Bipolar depression

One of the more difficult-to-diagnose but prevalent mental health conditions in the postpartum period is bipolar disorder. Once named "manic disorder," bipolar disorder manifests as type 1 with overtly manic states, while type 2 presents similarly to high-energy and low-energy states.[32] Linguistically and categorically, distinguishing between bipolar disorder and major depression with mixed features can be difficult.[32] However, it is thought that up to 20% of women with bipolar depression are diagnosed in the peripartum period.[33] Given this information, it is essential to glean the presence of a hypomanic or manic state in a patient who previously sought care for low mood and even anxiety.

Education About Treatment

Once the APC has identified a patient in the peripartum and screened using the PHQ-9, the GAD-7, or the EPDS, clinicians can probe the patient further and ask the appropriate questions that will allow them to tailor their education to the specific PMAD.

Patients should be educated about the risks and benefits of medication therapies and untreated mood disorders. Deciding to pursue medication therapy is a personal decision that only the patient can genuinely make in a shared decision-making model of care. Frequently, the mental health medication that a patient takes before pregnancy could work for the pregnant and lactating patient (**Fig. 1**). Using LactMed will help educate the patient about the relative infant dosing and known versus unknown risks of medication exposure to the baby.[34]

Non-pharmacologic Options

Patients should be educated that PMADs can be managed adjunctively or independently with psychological interventions, as exampled by the Mom-Me program based out of Philadelphia, PA.[35] This program conducted a peer support program focused on values, present moment awareness, understanding emotions, emotion regulation,

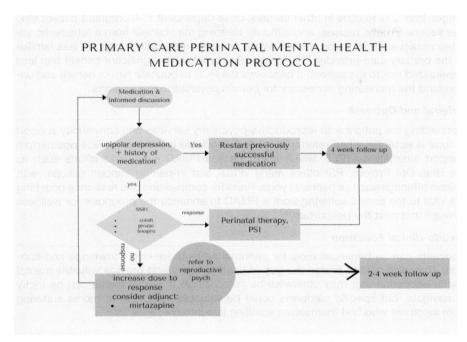

Fig. 1. Primary care perinatal mental health medication protocol.

acceptance, interpersonal effectiveness, and planful problem-solving with the goal of improving maternal functioning, and in turn symptoms of many PMADs.[35]

Pharmacologic Options

Medications may include serotonin reuptake inhibitors, serotonin and norepinephrine reuptake inhibitors, norepinephrine and dopamine reuptake inhibitors, as well as tricyclic antidepressants, benzodiazepines, and mood stabilizers.[36] New to the market and specific for PMAD treatment are neuroactive steroid gamma-aminobutyric acid (GABA) receptor modulators, once only available by intravenous infusion under the name Brexanolone, currently also available as a 14 day oral treatment under the name Zuranolone.[36] Patients should understand that, like many other medications, there may be some crossover through placental blood flow and breast milk for the breastfeeding patient.[34] However, for most medications, the exposure is limited, and the effects are minimal for the fetus or baby.[34] With this in mind, the parent must be given the appropriate education tailored to the individual's comfort level and medical needs.[34]

While some APCs may feel comfortable in medically managing PMADs with commonly prescribed antidepressants such as sertraline and escitalopram, it is essential to understand the variety of psychotropic medications that may be considered in the peripartum population with the correct risk–benefit discussion based on patient pregnancy status, breastfeeding status, and discussion of risk and benefit.[36]

For example, a postpartum patient at risk for bipolar depression with symptoms of severe depression and/or anxiety may benefit from considering a mood-stabilizing medication such as lamotrigine with a standing order titration or lithium if they are not breastfeeding.[36] Lamotrigine doses should, at a standard, be titrated to 200 mg over a 6 week course, with awareness for maternal milk serum lamotrigine transfer ranges from 2% to 30% in other studies, dose dependent.[34] A pregnant patient who has severe anxiety, nausea, and difficulty sleeping may benefit from a tetracyclic antidepressant such as mirtazapine.[36] While the latter medications may be less familiar to the primary care provider (PCP), they may be of more significant benefit and less generalized risk to the patient. It behooves the PCP to educate him or herself and understand the monitoring necessary for certain psychiatric medications.

Referral and Outreach

Connecting the patient with reproductive psychiatry services and community support groups is essential when referral is needed. Available resources include postpartum support international (PSI), which encompasses PMAD awareness efforts such as the Blue Dot Project. PSI offers many virtual and in-person support groups, with unique offerings such as perinatal yoga. Provider compassion and resilience coaching are vital to the parent suffering from a PMAD to enhance the prognosis for wellness through and past the peripartum.[37]

Pseudo-clinical Education

Podcasts can be beneficial tools for perinatal patients seeking knowledge and support. They also help to bridge the gap of health literacy and provide valuable mental health education that may otherwise be inaccessible.[38] Social media can be tricky to navigate, but specific platforms could be valuable resources to moms suffering from insomnia who find themselves scrolling late into the night.[39]

CLINICS CARE POINTS

- Perinatal mental health disorders can be safely managed in the primary care setting.
- The most commonly used antidepressants are selective serotonin reuptake inhibitors (SSRIs) but most patients do not understand how they work.
- It is a common misconception that the only SSRI available to pregnant and breastfeeding patients is sertraline.
- It is a common misconception that mood stabilizers, second-generation antipsychotics, norepinephrine, and dopamine reuptake inhibitors, and tricyclic antidepressants cannot be taken in pregnant and breastfeeding patients; however, many times, these medications are managed in concert with reproductive psychiatry consult.
- PSI makes available reproductive psychiatrists for providers who need consultation.

CASE STUDY
Postpartum Anxiety in a 25 Year Old White Woman

- A 25 year old white, assigned female at birth and identified as female presents to a community health center in rural Maryland with a *chief complaint of fatigue*.
- History of present illness.
    The patient has always felt exhausted since having her second child. When probed about her mood, she states she often feels irritable, on edge, and experiences difficulty sleeping. When she does fall asleep, she awakens through the night to check on her baby. She cannot stop worrying about something terrible happening to her baby and is afraid that he may stop breathing during his sleep. She tries to relax and enjoy a book during the baby's nap, but she cannot sit still and feels keyed up. She thought that she was doing much

better with managing symptoms of anxiety before her second child was born. She believed the anxious feelings would dissipate as the baby grew older, but now that he is 5 months old, she worries that this will never go away. She fears something is wrong with her and feels like her quality of life is very low, secondary to her feeling uneasy, worried, and nervous. She has been feeling this way nearly every day for the past 5 months. She had a form of these symptoms with her first child, but not this severe, and she never sought help in the past. She has never taken any medication for anxiety. She is currently breastfeeding. Her son is 5 months old and was born to a healthy pregnancy. The patient was followed by reproductive medicine throughout her pregnancy as she conceived with intrauterine insemination. She did not experience gestational hypertension or preeclampsia. She did not have gestational diabetes. She does report that she experienced heightened levels of anxiety during her pregnancy but attributed that to her 4 year old starting preschool. She is not currently in therapy. She has a sound support system at home and a safe relationship with her husband. She tries to walk outdoors but finds it challenging to find the time. She states that her son was born healthy at term, but the delivery was complicated by sustained bradycardia and a subsequent vacuum-assisted delivery. Baby's APGAR score was 8, but the patient had pictured a "golden hour" after birth, in which she would have 1 hour of uninterrupted skin-to-skin time with her newborn. This did not happen for reasons unknown to her. When asked, she stated this delivery did feel traumatic, although she did not feel this way with her daughter. She had laboratorys drawn 3 days before her visit today.

GAD-7: 14, PHQ-9: 4, ACE score: 0

Family History
 Mother: panic disorder, hypertension, hyperlipidemia
 Father: unknown
 Siblings: none
Medical History
 Binge eating disorder
Gynecologic and Obstetric History
 Uncomplicated pregnancy x2, vaginal delivery x2
 Gravida 2, 2-0-0-2
Social History
 Tobacco use: none
 Alcohol use: none
 Illicit drug use: none
Current Medications
 Prenatal multivitamin
 Sunflower lecithin
Vital Signs
 Blood pressure: 118/68; heart rate: 90; respiratory rate: 18; temperature: 36.8
 Weight: 143 lbs; height: 5 feet, 4 inches; body mass index: 24.5
Laboratory Values
Complete blood count (CBC): white blood cell 6.1, red blood cell 5.2, *hemoglobin 11.8, hematocrit 36.9*, MCV 78, mean corpuscular hemoglobin (MCH) 28, mean corpuscular hemoglobin concentration (MCHC) 32, red blood cell distribution width (RDW) 11.6, platelet 290, mean platelet volume 8.1

Complete metabolic panel (CMP): glucose 74, blood urea nitrogen (BUN) 10, creatinine 0.8, calcium 9, potassium 3.9, sodium 137, chloride 99, co2 24, albumin 3.9, alkaline phosphatase 40, total bilirubin 0.3, protein 6.0, alanine aminotransferase (ALT) 10, aspartate aminotransferase (AST) 12

Free thyroxine (T4) and thyroid stimulating hormone (TSH): free T4: 1.2, TSH 2.1

Imaging

None

- Clinical Questions

Do you have any further questions?

- *Has the patient ever experienced abnormally elevated moods?*
- *Has the patient experienced hallucinations or delusions?*
- *Has anyone in the family been diagnosed with bipolar disorder?*
- *Has the patient experienced thoughts of ending their own life?*
- *Has the patient experienced thoughts of harming themselves? Harming others?*
- *How does the patient feel about medication? About therapy?*

What is the assessment?

Generalized anxiety disorder in the postpartum patient

Borderline microcytic anemia

What is the plan of care?

Generalized anxiety disorder in the postpartum patient

- *Recommend cognitive behavioral therapy*
- *Recommend SSRI—potential options to consider: sertraline, escitalopram, citalopram, fluoxetine, paroxetine*
- *Chosen SSRI in this case: fluoxetine*

Rationale: The patient has a history of binge eating disorder, and fluoxetine is also Food and Drug Administration approved for binge eating disorder.

Patient education

In combination with psychotherapy, antidepressant medications can be beneficial to combat anxiety symptoms. SSRIs are a type of antidepressant. Common side effects of SSRIs include stomach upset within the first few weeks, libido shifts, and weight shifts. All patients who are prescribed SSRIs should be cautioned that if they experience suicidal ideation, they should immediately stop the medication and seek medical care. However, this is a rare occurrence in adults with unipolar depression. All SSRIs taken by the breastfeeding parent are present in breast milk. In studies thus far, the amount of SSRI is typically very low to undetectable in infant serum. When deciding to pursue medication treatment, weighing the benefits against the risks is important. At the same time, I believe the benefit outweighs the risk in your particular case, as a mentally healthy parent is essential for the baby's health, in my opinion, more so than the minute risk of neonatal side effects. Rare but possible side effects of SSRI neonatal effect would be jitteriness, difficulty sleeping, feeding problems, or somnolence, which should prompt the mother to see neonatal assessment by their pediatrician.[20] Fluoxetine is a longer acting antidepressant and may take more time to notice positive effects. As long as you do not experience any adverse reaction to the drug, I would recommend continuing daily until our follow-up appointment. Follow-up is recommended in 4 to 6 weeks to assess response.

SUMMARY

When the primary care APC helps parents advocate for their mental health, they help not only bridge the gap between specialty care and primary care accessibility but also elicit positive downstream health outcomes for the birthing parent, baby, and family. PMADs often go unrecognized, but the impact on the patient and their family stretches far outside the peripartum. APCs can reach these patients across a diverse set of health care settings, offer treatment, and connect the patient with the appropriate resources for whole body and mind care. Thorough history-taking and proper utilization of screening tools will allow the APC to offer medical management. Foundational knowledge in psychopharmacology can be applied across the peripartum, and gestalt of referral can be used to cultivate best practices in the peripartum mental health arena.

FUTURE DIRECTIONS

Further research needs to be done to learn how to best incorporate mental health in primary care for the perinatal patient. Current limitations include time and provider familiarity with pathologic mental health states adversely affecting the birthing parent and baby and how best to support the family unit as a primary care provider.

CLINICS CARE POINTS

- While screening tools are imperative to identify perinatal mental health disorders, they are just the beginning.
- Many commonly prescribed anti-depressants and anti-anxiety medications can be safely prescribed in the primary care setting in conjunction with the obstetric team, but educating the patient is key to implementing a successful pharmacotherapeutic treatment plan.
- Listening to the patient is the first and most critical component in creating the best plan of care for the mental health of the pregnant and postpartum patient.

DISCLOSURE

The author has no relevant financial or nonfinancial relationships to disclose.

REFERENCES

1. Byatt N, Masters GA, Twyman J, et al. Building obstetric provider capacity to address perinatal depression through online training. J Womens Health (Larchmt) 2021 Oct;30(10):1386–94. Epub 2021 Apr 9. PMID: 33835884; PMCID: PMC8590156.
2. Howard LM, Khalifeh H. Perinatal mental health: a review of progress and challenges. World Psychiatr 2020;19(3):313–27.
3. Pokharel A, Philip S, Khound M, et al. Mental illness stigma among perinatal women in low- and middle-income countries: early career psychiatrists' perspective. Front Psychiatry 2023;14:1283715. Published 2023 Dec 5.
4. Silverwood V, Bullock L, Jordan J, et al. Non-pharmacological interventions for the management of perinatal anxiety in primary care: a meta-review of systematic reviews. BJGP Open 2023;7(3). https://doi.org/10.3399/BJGPO.2023.0022. BJGPO.2023.0022.
5. Orchard ER, Rutherford HJV, Holmes AJ, et al. Matrescence: lifetime impact of motherhood on cognition and the brain. Trends Cogn Sci 2023;27(3):302–16.

6. Kirkpatrick CE, Lee S. Comparisons to picture-perfect motherhood: How Instagram's idealized portrayals of motherhood affect new mothers' well-being. Comput Human Behav 2022;137:107417.

7. Thompson HM, Clement AM, Ortiz R, et al. Community engagement to improve access to healthcare: a comparative case study to advance implementation science for transgender health equity. Int J Equity Health 2022;21(1):104. Published 2022 Jul 31.

8. Alvarado C.S., Cassidy D., Orgera K., et al., Polling spotlight: understanding the experiences of LGBTQ+ birthing people, 2022, Center For Health Justice, Available at: https://www.aamchealthjustice.org/news/polling/lgbtq-birth (Accessed 14 January 2024).

9. Mughal S, Azhar Y, Siddiqui W. Postpartum depression. In: StatPearls. Treasure Island (FL): StatPearls Publishing; 2024. Available at: https://www.ncbi.nlm.nih.gov/books/NBK519070/.

10. Chin K, Wendt A, Bennett IM, et al. Suicide and Maternal Mortality. Curr Psychiatry Rep 2022;24(4):239–75.

11. Pregnancy risk assessment monitoring system. Centers for Disease Control and Prevention; 2023. Available at: https://www.cdc.gov/prams/index.htm. [Accessed 14 January 2024].

12. Garcia ER, Yim IS. A systematic review of concepts related to women's empowerment in the perinatal period and their associations with perinatal depressive symptoms and premature birth. BMC Pregnancy Childbirth 2017;17(2):347.

13. Witt WP, Wisk LE, Cheng ER, et al. Preconception mental health predicts pregnancy complications and adverse birth outcomes: a national population-based study. Matern Child Health J 2012;16(7):1525–41.

14. Nuyts T, Van Haeken S, Crombag N, et al. "Nobody Listened". Mothers' E=experiences and needs regarding professional support prior to their admission to an infant mental health day clinic. Int J Environ Res Public Health 2021;18(20):10917. Published 2021 Oct 17.

15. Hernandez ND, Francis S, Allen M, et al. Prevalence and predictors of symptoms of Perinatal Mood and anxiety Disorders among a sample of Urban Black Women in the South. Matern Child Health J 2022;26(4):770–7.

16. Estriplet T, Morgan I, Davis K, et al. Black Perinatal Mental Health: Prioritizing Maternal Mental Health to Optimize Infant Health and Wellness. Front Psychiatr 2022;13. https://doi.org/10.3389/fpsyt.2022.807235.

17. Cho H, Lee K, Choi E, et al. Association between social support and postpartum depression. Sci Rep 2022;12(1):3128.

18. Pohl AL, Crockford SK, Blakemore M, et al. A comparative study of autistic and non-autistic women's experience of motherhood. Mol Autism 2020;11(1):3. Published 2020 Jan 6.

19. Beydoun HA, Al-Sahab B, Beydoun MA, et al. Intimate partner violence as a risk factor for postpartum depression among Canadian women in the Maternity Experience Survey. Ann Epidemiol 2010;20(8):575–83.

20. Pranckeviciene A, Saudargiene A, Gecaite-Stonciene J, et al. Validation of the patient health questionnaire-9 and the generalized anxiety disorder-7 in Lithuanian student sample. PLoS One 2022;17(1):e0263027. Published 2022 Jan 27.

21. Bodenlos KL, Maranda L, Deligiannidis KM. Comparison of the use of the epds-3 vs. Epds-10 to identify women at risk for peripartum depression [3k]. Obstet Gynecol 2016;127(Supplement 1):89S–90S.

22. Vanderkruik R, Raffi E, Freeman MP, et al. Perinatal depression screening using smartphone technology: Exploring uptake, engagement and future directions

for the MGH Perinatal Depression Scale (MGHPDS). PLoS One 2021;16(9): e0257065.

23. Webb R, Uddin N, Ford E, et al. Barriers and facilitators to implementing perinatal mental health care in health and social care settings: a systematic review. Lancet Psychiatr 2021;8(6):521–34.

24. Galea LAM, Frokjaer VG. Perinatal depression: embracing variability toward better treatment and outcomes. Neuron 2019;102(1):13–6.

25. Garapati J, Jajoo S, Aradhya D, et al. Postpartum Mood Disorders: Insights into Diagnosis, Prevention, and Treatment. Cureus 2023;15(7):e42107.

26. Baby blues and postpartum depression: mood disorders and pregnancy. 2023. Available at: https://www.hopkinsmedicine.org/health/wellness-and-prevention/postpartum-mood-disorders-what-new-moms-need-to-know. [Accessed 12 April 2024].

27. Perinatal Mental Health Training, Webinar presented at: Postpartum Support International, Available at: https://www.postpartum.net/professionals/frontline-provider-trainings/. (Accessed 20 April 2024).

28. Iranpour S, Kheirabadi GR, Esmaillzadeh A, et al. Association between sleep quality and postpartum depression. J Res Med Sci 2016;21:110. PMID: 28250787; PMCID: PMC5322694.

29. Puyané M, Subirà S, Torres A, et al. Personality traits as a risk factor for postpartum depression: A systematic review and meta-analysis. J Affect Disord 2022;298:577–89.

30. Center for Substance Abuse Treatment (US). Trauma-informed care in behavioral health services. Rockville (MD): Substance Abuse and Mental Health Services Administration (US); 2014 (Treatment Improvement Protocol (TIP) Series, No. 57.) Exhibit 1.3-4, DSM-5 Diagnostic Criteria for PTSD. Available at: https://www.ncbi.nlm.nih.gov/books/NBK207191/box/part1_ch3.box16/.

31. Kranenburg L, Lambregtse-van den Berg M, Stramrood C. Traumatic childbirth experience and childbirth-related post-traumatic stress disorder (PTSD): a contemporary overview. Int J Environ Res Public Health 2023;20(4):2775.

32. Bipolar disorder - national institute of mental health(Nimh). Available at: https://www.nimh.nih.gov/health/topics/bipolar-disorder. [Accessed 12 April 2024].

33. MGH Center for Women's Mental Health. Prevalence of bipolar disorder and bipolar-spectrum mood episodes during pregnancy and the postpartum period in perinatal women - MGH center for women's mental health. MGH Center for Women's Mental Health - Perinatal & Reproductive Psychiatry at Mass General Hospital. 2022. Available at: https://womensmentalhealth.org/posts/perinatal-obsessive-compulsive-related-disorder. [Accessed 14 January 2024].

34. National Institute of Health. Drugs and Lactation Database (LactMed®) Internet. Bethesda (MD): National Institute of Child Health and Human Development; 2006. Available at: https://www.ncbi.nlm.nih.gov/books/NBK501922/.

35. Grunberg VA, Geller PA, Durham K, et al. Motherhood and Me (Mom-Me): The Development of an Acceptance-Based Group for Women with Postpartum Mood and Anxiety Symptoms. J Clin Med 2022;11(9):2345.

36. Perinatal mental health psychopharmacology. Postpartum Support International (PSI). January 12. 2024. Available at: https://www.postpartum.net/professionals/certificate-trainings/psychopharmacology/. [Accessed 13 January 2024].

37. Saharoy R, Potdukhe A, Wanjari M, et al. postpartum depression and maternal care: exploring the complex effects on mothers and infants. Cureus 2023;15(7): e41381.

38. Caoilte NÓ, Lambert S, Murphy R, et al. Podcasts as a tool for enhancing mental health literacy: An investigation of mental health-related podcasts. Mental Health & Prevention 2023;30:200285.
39. Moon RY, Mathews A, Oden R, et al. Mothers' Perceptions of the Internet and Social Media as Sources of Parenting and Health Information: Qualitative Study. J Med Internet Res 2019;21(7):e14289.

Assessing the Effectiveness of Patient Education

Felix Alvelo, MPAS, PA-C[a], Susan M. Salahshor, PhD, PA-C, DFAAPA[b],*,
Jordan Beckley, MPAS, PA-C[c]

KEYWORDS

- Patient education • Health education • Health belief model • Learning theory model
- Intervention planning model • PEMAT • Assessment tool • Health care barriers

KEY POINTS

- This article describes the theoretic models that underpin patient education.
- It discusses the current assessment tools used in patient education and explains implementation.
- It discusses the challenges and barriers to patient education in health care.
- It explains the impact of the effectiveness of patient education.

INTRODUCTION

Poor health literacy is linked to increased mortality rates and adverse medical outcomes in patients.[1] Health promotion and disease prevention are the end goal of any clinician. As medicine becomes more transparent and information becomes more accessible, today's patients actively seek education and ways to manage their illnesses.[2] They are turning to open-sourced information, especially when they have unanswered questions from their clinicians.[2] Patient education is one of the best tools to provide a change in our patients' care, which is why clinicians remain stewards of information delivery. Every clinician should assess patient education and content delivery to determine effectiveness. This article discusses the theoretic foundations of patient education, its establishment, and its transformation over the years. It examines modern patient education challenges, such as limited appointment times and health literacy with diverse populations. The article concludes with current evidence-based assessment tools and future directions to improve patient education.

[a] Mid Valley Clinic & Hospital, 529 Jasmine Street, Omak, WA 98841, USA; [b] Ottawa University, 4370 West 109 Street #200, Overland Park, KS 66211, USA; [c] CVS Minute Clinic, 6 DuPont Circle Northwest, Washington, DC 20036, USA
* Corresponding author.
E-mail address: Susan.salahshor@ottawa.edu

Physician Assist Clin 9 (2024) 589–599
https://doi.org/10.1016/j.cpha.2024.05.010
2405-7991/24/Published by Elsevier Inc.

physicianassistant.theclinics.com

BACKGROUND AND CONTEXT

Patient education is a fundamental component of patient health and successful outcomes. The communication among clinicians, patients, and their caregivers in a structured or unstructured manner should follow a logical sequence to enhance understanding.[3] The medical culture trend in the 1960s defined patients as passive; therefore, education was not frequently part of the comprehensive health visit.[4] This would gradually change in the 1970s, soon after the Lalonde Report in Canada.

The 1974 Lalonde Report considered health went beyond traditional biological medical care and emphasized the importance of socioeconomic factors.[5] During the same time in Europe, the Netherlands was one of the leaders in developing educational programs in patient care, defining the role of patient education in primary care, and creating programs that assess its effectiveness in hospitals.[4] These chains of events led to today's advancements.

PATIENT EDUCATION LANDSCAPE

The literature showed that from the 1800s to the 1900s, physicians and other therapeutic professionals were viewed as the teachers and clinicians of health in medicine.[6] Patients were instructed about their health and were not expected to participate in decision-making.[6] The medical community and patients alike accepted that the healthy lifestyle was physician led. However, this began to change.

Over time, numerous factors influenced patients' rights, including the civil rights and women's movement and consumer and patient rights advocacy. Organizations and professional groups began to increase their focus on patient education, including the veteran administration, the Centers for Disease Control and Prevention (CDC), the Food and Drug Administration, physician training groups, and health insurers.[3] The nursing profession incorporated diabetes education, and public health professionals paved the way by changing laws.[3] The evolution of patient education from a clinician to a patient-driven one was born.

Health Belief Model

More effective patient education uses models from social psychology to help determine how to educate patients best, such as the Health Belief Model (HBM).[7] HBM was created in the 1950s by social psychologists after recognizing that clinicians lacked considering the whole patient and disease management and prevention.[8] In the 1950s, the components of HBM were (1) perceived susceptibility, (2) perceived severity, (3) perceived benefits and costs, and (4) motivation (**Table 1**).[8,9] The HBM addressed the ineffectiveness of managing diseases, such as tuberculosis, patients' unwillingness to accept vaccines, and dental hygiene concerns.[7]

Table 1 Health belief model components	
Component	**Question Asked**
Perceived Susceptibility	*What is the risk of getting the disease?*
Perceived Severity	*How bad will the disease and its symptoms be?*
Perceived Benefits and Costs	*How much does it cost (time, resources, money, people)? Based on the clinician's recommendations, what are the benefits of managing my condition?*
Motivation	*What is the impact on my daily life?*

Learning Theory Model

Patient education evolved from telling patients what to do to teaching patients about their conditions and addressing beneficial behaviors so the patient can make more informed decisions. It supports health beyond clinicians.[9] The evolution includes the delivery modes. Patients communicated in 3 modes: (1) verbally by clinicians, (2) paper handouts, and (3) Web sites.[10]

Clinicians should focus on communicating information to patients using the patients' lived experiences and direct communication. There are 5 components of the learning theory when providing patient education: (1) reinforcement, (2) feedback, (3) individualism, (4) facilitation, and (5) relevance (**Fig. 1**).[9] Reinforcement is complimenting the patient on positive outcomes after education. Feedback tells the patients how their behavior impacts the disease or condition. Individualism recognizes the patients' social, environmental, and cultural educational experiences. Facilitation asks questions while considering the patients' views on the disease or condition. Relevance asks, "How does the outcome impact the patient's life?"

Intervention Planning Model

Researchers recommended 6 steps to assess the effectiveness of an intervention: what will influence behavior change, what is the benchmark aim to determine the education-changed behavior, select a proven method to affect behavioral change, create education resources to address the behavior change needed, consider, and list potential barriers to achieving the benchmark, and reassess the intervention undertaken.[9]

The intervention planning model was intended to make patient education effective for the patient and health profession. The model is composed of 5 steps:

1. Identify the problem and the need.
2. List the relevant behaviors.
3. Outline what influences these behaviors.
4. Create an intervention and use it.
5. Assess whether the intervention is effective.[9]

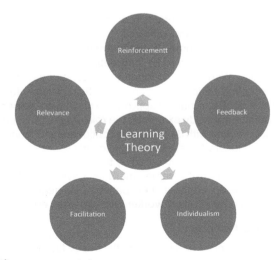

Fig. 1. Learning theory components.

The most critical components are the patient's active role in the shared decision-making process and buy-in to the education. Some authors proposed that patients must actively participate in the decision tree through education in multiple delivery modes.[11] The theoretic models offer opportunities to improve patient education, but challenges remain, such as patients may struggle due to cultural, language, and trust barriers.

CHALLENGES AND CONSIDERATIONS

Patient education remains fraught with challenges that require multifaceted strategies and dedicated attention from clinicians. Patient education is an indispensable aspect of modern health care, ensuring that patients are informed, empowered, and capable of making decisions that align with their health goals. Barriers and challenges can hinder the process, including health literacy levels, clinician time constraints, cultural and linguistic misunderstandings, and lack of trust in the health care delivery system.

Health Literacy

Health literacy is at the forefront of barriers in patient education. To access patient education, prior knowledge, motivation, and competencies are needed to make judgments in everyday life concerning health care, disease prevention, and health promotion.[12] Patients with low health literacy skills have insufficient reading, writing, and numeracy skills for practical education in the health context.[12,13] A systematic review indicated that low health literacy consistently correlates with increased hospital admissions, a higher reliance on emergency services, a reduced capacity to administer medications appropriately, challenges in understanding labels and health-related messages, and a decline in general health and an increased mortality rate in older patients.[1] Research has also indicated that clinicians frequently fail to identify health literacy challenges in working-age adults who can converse fluently in the prevalent language.[14] It is imperative for us as clinicians to recognize the varying health literacy levels in our patients. By doing so, we can tailor patient education to an individual's unique needs and perspective, ensuring a more personalized and practical health care experience.

Time Constraints

Shared decision-making and patient education get compromised due to an unequal clinician–patient supply and demand ratio, clinicians having limited time to spend with each patient, and a high volume of appointments. Rushed appointments may result in incomplete information shared or information presented too quickly for patients to understand fully. With these constraints, evidence has shown that detailed shared decision-making and patient education are difficult to maintain; therefore, clinicians may default to a decision-making approach with little-to-no personalization for the patient.[15] An experimental study examined the role of time pressure on adherence to guidelines in clinical practice with 34 general practitioners and found that under time pressure, General practitioners (GPs) asked significantly fewer questions concerning presenting symptoms than the ones indicated by the guidelines and conducted a less thorough clinical examination. At the same time, they gave less advice on lifestyle.[16] Clinicians need more time to educate their patients, or health care organizations should implement having a health care worker who provides education.

Cultural and Linguistic Differences

Cultural and linguistic differences and other health literacy factors can pose considerable challenges to patient education. According to the Institute of Medicine (IOM), health literacy should consider the context of language and culture.[17] Comprehension of health information is deeply rooted in one's linguistic abilities and cultural perspectives. Crucial health information is missed if there is a misalignment between clinicians' language and patients' understanding. Cultural beliefs influence perceptions of illness, health behaviors, and interactions with health care systems. Recognizing and addressing the interplay between language, culture, and health literacy ensure that health care information is accessible, relevant, and effective for diverse populations, leading to better health outcomes and patient-centered care.

Lack of Trust in the Health Care System

Historical and individual experiences can lead patients to mistrust clinicians. When trust is lacking, the patient might be reluctant to believe or act upon the information provided. Given historical injustices and systemic biases in health care, building trust with specific patient groups may require extra effort. Transgenerational trauma can hinder the establishment of a comprehensive and trusting patient–clinician relationship.[18] For example, since the introduction of slavery in the American colonies, black individuals have faced limited and subpar health care access, leading to poorer health outcomes.[18] Evidence has shown that these deliberately orchestrated disparities benefit the health care systems.[18] These historical factors continue to contribute to various populations' mistrust.

Ethical Considerations

Addressing the challenges in patient education brings to the forefront several ethical considerations and dilemmas. Ethical health care is built on the 4 biomedical principles of autonomy, beneficence, non-maleficence, and justice.[19] These principles occasionally conflict when providing patient education.[19] Patients have the right to make decisions about their health care even when it does not align with the clinicians' perceptions of non-maleficence.

Biomedical Principles

Informed decisions require appropriate education by clinicians. However, the challenge arises when patients refuse necessary treatments due to a lack of understanding. The ethical dilemma is balancing respecting the patients' autonomy with the need to provide beneficial care. While clinicians aim to do what is best for patients (beneficence), they must avoid causing harm (non-maleficence). If patients do not fully grasp their condition's severity due to insufficient education and fail to follow treatment protocols, it may cause harm. Yet, pushing too hard to ensure compliance might infringe on their autonomy. Addressing these challenges requires empathy, cultural competency, and a deep understanding of medical ethics and individual patients' needs. By recognizing and thoughtfully navigating these ethical considerations, health care clinicians can ensure a more holistic and ethically sound approach to patient education.[19]

Cultural and Diversity Considerations

Successful patient education must be culturally competent, attuned to diversity, and consistently evaluated for accuracy and relevance. Its effectiveness should be assessed from a dual perspective. When disseminating information to patients, it is beneficial to circle or highlight significant points rather than merely providing a patient with a pamphlet or handout. Personalizing the material and employing the "teach-back" or feedback methods during patient education can also ensure the patient's comprehension and allow them to ask questions in real time. Standard post-care surveys can also enable patients to provide feedback on their care, helping clinicians enhance specific areas. From a system and clinician standpoint, effectiveness assessments necessitate clinicians to commit to ongoing education and be receptive to adjusting educational tactics based on the distinct needs of diverse groups. By adopting such practices, the health care sector can guarantee that patient education transcends mere information dissemination, becoming a conduit for understanding and mutual respect.

Patient education should be diverse and adaptable. There is a linkage between the effectiveness of patient education and patients' diverse cultural backgrounds and individual experiences. A "one-size-fits-all" approach fails to recognize the intricacies of diverse populations. The nuances of culture and diversity play a significant role in shaping beliefs, attitudes, and behaviors related to health. Thus, exploring these factors is pivotal to ensuring that patient education is informative, resonant, and impactful. To determine the most effective method to convey information tailored to individual patients, asking them about their preferences and learning styles is essential. Whether through written materials, audio recordings, instructional videos, a step-by-step approach, or even a trained peer educator, it is vital to utilize various tools to meet the patients where they are and ensure their understanding and engagement.[20]

When assessing the impact of the effectiveness of patient education, first, look at cultural beliefs. Cultural health beliefs affect how people think and feel about their health and health problems, when and from whom they seek care, and how they respond to recommendations for lifestyle change, health care interventions, and treatment adherence.[21] Cultures differ in their communication styles, the meaning of words and gestures, and discussion about the body, health, and illness.[21] Direct communication about health concerns varies based on cultural norms. Patients might avoid discussing specific topics due to cultural taboos or stigmas. Clinicians must understand and respect these preferences for effective education while ensuring the patient receives the necessary information.

Consider what role family and communities play in a patient's culture and their ability to use their patient education. In these contexts, patient education might need to involve a broader group rather than focusing solely on the individual. For example, Middle Eastern cultures have large extended families that are heavily involved in patient care.[22] If patients require family members' input in decision-making, they should identify one responsible family member to communicate with the clinician to ensure proper and structured family involvement to help improve patient care.

BEST PRACTICES AND STRATEGIES

The assessment of patient education material aids clinicians in fortifying their patient-to-clinician communication and vital care instructions. There must be a standard assessment to understand the effectiveness of medical education.

Patient Education Material Assessment Tool

The Patient Education Material Assessment Tool (PEMAT) was created by the Department of Health and Human Services as a national action plan to improve overall health literacy in the United States.[23] It is a universal tool created for clinicians and the public.[23] Its systemic method evaluates patients with 2 main domains: understandability and actionability (**Table 2**). Understandability is the effectiveness of how patients absorb and present critical messages.[23] Actionability is the effectiveness of how patients can translate obtained information to personal change.[23]

Table 2
Comparison of PEMAT versions

Versions	Assessment Material	Understandability Questions	Actionability Questions
PEMAT-P	(Print) Pamphlets, brochures	17 items	7 items
PEMAT-A/V	(Audiovisual) Videos, multimedia	13 items	4 items

As seen in **Table 2**, there are 2 versions of the PEMAT, print and audiovisual. PEMAT-P is for specific printable pamphlets, brochures, and physical material. This type incorporates 17 questions expanding the domain of understandability by assessing the organization of information, white space, and visual illustrations.[24] The actionability domain within PEMAT-P uses 7 questions to expand on tangible tools, such as planners, checklists, and simple calculations.[24] Example questions and format are illustrated in **Table 3**, which guides the user in evaluating the domains of understandability and actionability.

PEMAT-A/V is for specific audiovisual material that includes multimedia and videos. Although this version has comparable questions to PEMAT-P, PEMAT A/V omits certain aspects of assessments seen in the printable version to account for text screen size, audio speed, and sound. PMAT-A/V has 13 understandability questions and 4 actionability questions in its design.[23]

PEMAT-P and PEMAT A/V are answered by 2 choices, "agree," equating to 1 point, and "disagree," which is 0 point, as seen in **Table 3**.[23] Questions include a "not applicable" option as well. The clinician should total the scores, divide by the number of questions, and multiply by 100, resulting in a percentage. Higher percentages indicate the most effective material.

Institutions, including the National Institute of Health (NIH), the CDC, and the Agency for Healthcare Research and Quality, use the PEMAT. The National Cancer Institute focused on the interrater reliability of PEMAT by assessing raters and disbursing 110 patient education materials to patients and caregivers.[24] PEMAT had a high interrater reliable rating across all questions, making it an effective assessment tool.[24]

Although PEMAT is an effective tool for patient education, it has limitations. PEMAT does not assess information accuracy, comprehensiveness, and reading level.[23] Clinicians evaluate and review the accuracy and comprehensiveness of the results. At times, these educational materials include an abundance of jargon. The average

Table 3
Example questions with answer format

Item #	Item	Response Option	Rating
Understandability			
1	The material's purpose is clear.	Disagree = 0, Agree = 1	
2	The material uses every day and known language.	Disagree = 0, Agree = 1	
Actionability			
1	The material defines actions for the reader.	Disagree = 0, Agree = 1	
2	The material provides simple instructions.	Disagree = 0, Agree = 1	

American reads at an 8 or 9 grade level.[25] The NIH and the American Medical Association (AMA) encourage patient education material at a sixth grade level.[25] As a result, readability assessment tools are widely used in conjunction with the PEMAT for patient education.

Simple Measure of Gobbledygook (SMOG) is a handwritten, readability assessment tool. SMOG helps assessors determine patient information grade level by counting 10 sentences of a document from beginning, middle, and end.[25] Then, the assessor calculates all the words with more than 3 syllables.[25] The more complex words correlate to higher grade-level writing. The Flesch–Kincaid grade level (FKGL) method is another widely used readability assessment tool. FK is a computerized assessment tool added to Microsoft Word spelling and grammar checks that identify syllables in the text.[25] A readability statistic is calculated once the document is put through the spell-check feature.

CASE STUDY EXAMPLE

Applying PEMAT and readability tools such as SMOG and FKGL improves the quality of patient education, thus increasing patient communication, lowering patient anxiety, and improving medical outcomes.[26] An article focusing on online material related to vocal cord leukoplakia, PEMAT, SMOG, and FKGL assessed patient education on 50 Web sites by determining the quality of understandability, actionability, and readability.[27] Web sites in this study included institutions such as Mayo Clinic, Mount Sinai, Cornell, John Hopkins Medicine, and Columbia.[27] This study concluded that none of the Web sites met the AMA and NIH recommendations of reading levels below sixth grade.[27] The Web sites were between 12 and 16 grade levels, with understandability and actionability scores of 73% and 13%, respectively.[27] In conclusion, online material on vocal cord leukoplakia requires a higher level of reading, creating lower patient understandability and not adequately outlining discrete steps, producing poor actionability.[26]

Large government entities such as the National Center of Quality Improvement and the Institute of Health Care Improvement promote the adoption and implementation of patient-centered care.[28] Recently, the United States has applied regulations and incentives to encourage clinicians to create clinical summaries so patients can access them through electronic medical records (EMRs) to improve education.[28] This study applied PEMAT, SMOG, and FKGL to assess the characteristics of clinical summaries from EHR in 13 practices.[28] The study found that median PEMAT scores demonstrated 65% for understandability and 78% for actionability[28] (2016). The average median reading level for FKGL was ninth grade, and SMOG was 11th.[28] Clinical summaries were fair in suitability, understandability, and actionability while requiring high reading levels with small font sizes.[28]

FUTURE DIRECTIONS AND OPPORTUNITIES

As leaders in the medical field, clinicians need to acknowledge how to communicate effectively with patients. In doing so, clinicians need to understand patient education assessment tools and apply that knowledge to patient education materials. The assessment of patient education continues to evolve to meet the demand for improved patient outcomes. Health care is moving toward a more inclusive environment.

Assessment tools like PEMAT focus on understandability and actionability but do not elaborate on culture. The Health Education Assessment tool instituted by the NIH has formulated a patient education assessment tool that incorporates the PEMAT and cultural relevance.[29] This tool does not just determine whether materials are easy to read, but it also keeps cultural considerations in mind.[29] For example, does the educational material supply understandable examples of activities, foods, language, and images to specific ethnic groups, and are stereotypes avoided.[29] Although cultural relevance assessment tools are lacking, future development promises changes.

Today, technology is starting to be an ever-changing patient education tool. Artificial intelligence (AI) will be intertwined with health care in some capacity in the future.[30] Even though AI still has limitations, generative pretrained transformer (GPT) has already been introduced in the health care setting, specifically in radiology.[30] ChatGPT is a data set of text that can produce natural verbiage.[30] AI may have a role in the accuracy and efficiency of radiologic imaging, which can aid in diagnostics.[30] As patients have more accessibility to their EMRs, translating medical language becomes an effective patient education tool. GPT is the median where language translation and test summarization provide patients with knowledge and understanding.[30] Future software programmed into patient education assessment tools adds understanding of medical information.

RECOMMENDATIONS

The current trend in medical information is transparency. Patients have easier access to their health records through online patient portals, allowing them to see medical information before they are interpreted.[2] Health care organizations incentivized clinicians to complete clinical summaries for patients' reference.[28] Consumer accessibility to medical information has improved outcomes and experiences and has lower costs.[2] Future research to determine how clinical summaries and uninterpreted medical results are helpful to patient health outcomes and how patients will respond to these results without proper education is warranted. Clinicians should follow AMA and NIH recommendations on readability at a sixth grade level.

Future efforts should include the use of technological tools to increase understanding. Technology tools incorporate patient education models based on the patients, their cultural backgrounds, social determinants of health, view of health care, and comfort levels. Intertwined with technology and models is the ability of patients to utilize recommendations and manage their medical conditions.

Educational materials and communication methods should align with each patient's health literacy, cultural background, and language needs. This customization can involve creating straightforward visual aids, simplifying language for more precise understanding, and providing resources in multiple languages. Such an approach ensures that information is accessible and understandable to all patients, regardless of their background.

Effective patient education to patients and understanding where to get this information is essential. MedLine Plus is one example. MedLine Plus is part of the NIH and is the world's largest medical library information resource for patients and families, and it is free to the public.[31] It includes deeper details of medications, system-based health topics, laboratory interpretations, and even healthy recipes.[31] Health topics include over 1,000 diseases and illnesses with over 4,000 medical encyclopedia articles.[31] Medline Plus has implemented patient assessment tools for more digestible patient education.

In addition, establishing a patient-centered approach is critical to overcoming distrust in the health care system. By focusing on these elements, clinicians can build trust, encouraging patients to take a more active role in their health care journey. This involves clear communication, respecting patients' autonomy in their care decisions, and ensuring consistent follow-up.

SUMMARY

Patient education is part of the delivery of safe and effective patient care. Patients continue to be increasingly engaged in gathering information about their conditions. Clinicians must evaluate the models, tools, and evidence-based data to provide adequate, appropriate, and culturally relevant patient education. Integrating patients, clinicians, and education is now required for better outcomes.

CLINICS CARE POINTS

- Clinicians should consider social factors when educating patients.
- Application of PEMAT, SMOG, and FKGL and how they impact patient assessment should be kept in mind.
- Clinicians should consider cultural and linguistic abilities in patient assessment with PEMAT and cultural relevance.

DISCLOSURE

The authors have nothing to disclose.

REFERENCES

1. Berkman ND, Sheridan SL, Donahue KE, et al. Low health literacy and health outcomes: an updated systematic review. Ann Intern Med 2011;155(2):97–107.
2. Johnson AM, Brimhall AS, Johnson ET, et al. A systematic review of the effectiveness of patient education through patient portals. JAMIA Open 2023;6(1): ooac085. Published 2023 Jan 18.
3. Bartlett EE. Historical glimpses of patient education in the United States. Patient Educ Couns 1986;8(2):135–49.
4. Hoving C, Visser A, Mullen PD, et al. A history of patient education by health professionals in Europe and North America: from authority to shared decision making education. Patient Educ Couns 2010;78(3):275–81.
5. Glouberman S, Millar J. Evolution of the determinants of Health, health policy, and Health Information Systems in Canada. Am J Public Health 2003;93(3):388–92.
6. Breslow L. Patient education in historical perspective. Bull N Y Acad Med 1985; 61(2):115–22. Available at: https://www.ncbi.nlm.nih.gov/pmc/articles/PMC 1911823/. [Accessed 10 December 2023].
7. Bellamy R. An introduction to patient education: Theory and practice. Med Teach 2004;26(4):359–65.
8. Becker MH. The Health Belief Model and sick role behavior. Health Educ Monogr 1974;2(4):409–19.
9. Janz NK, Becker MH. The Health Belief Model: a decade later. Health Educ Q 1984;11(1):1–47. https://doi.org/10.1177/109019818401100101.
10. Van den Borne HW. The patient from receiver of information to informed decision-maker. Patient Educ Couns 1998;34(2):89–102.
11. Gruman J, Rovner MH, French ME, et al. From patient education to patient engagement: implications for field of patient education. Patient Educ Couns 2010;78(3):350–6.
12. Wittink H, Oosterhaven J. Patient education and health literacy. Musculoskelet Sci Pract 2018;38:120–7. https://doi.org/10.1016/j.msksp.2018.06.004.

13. Easton P, Entwistle VA, Williams B. Health in the 'hidden population' of people with low literacy. A systematic review of the literature. BMC Public Health 2010;10:459. Published 2010 Aug 5.

14. Caverly TJ, Hayward RA. Dealing with the Lack of Time for Detailed Shared Decision-making in Primary Care: Everyday Shared Decision-making. J Gen Intern Med 2020;35(10):3045–9.

15. Tsiga E, Panagopoulou E, Sevdalis N, et al. The influence of time pressure on adherence to guidelines in primary care: an experimental study. BMJ Open 2013;3:e002700. Published 2013 Apr 11.

16. Andrulis DP, Brach C. Integrating literacy, culture, and language to improve health care quality for diverse populations. Am J Health Behav 2007;31(Suppl 1):S122–33.

17. Miller F, Miller P. Transgenerational trauma and trust restoration. AMA J Ethics 2021;23(6):E480–6. Published 2021 Jun 1.

18. Olejarczyk JP, Young M. Patient Rights and Ethics. In: StatPearls. Treasure Island (FL): StatPearls Publishing; 2022. Available at: https://pubmed.ncbi.nlm.nih.gov/30855863/.

19. Use Health Education Material Effectively: Tool 12. AHRQ. Available at: https://www.ahrq.gov/health-literacy/improve/precautions/tool12.html. [Accessed 27 December 2023].

20. Varkey B. Principles of clinical ethics and their application to practice. Med Princ Pract 2021;30(1):17–28.

21. Institute of Medicine (US) Committee on Health Literacy. In: Nielsen-Bohlman L, Panzer AM, Kindig DA, editors. Health literacy: a prescription to end confusion. Washington (DC): National Academies Press (US); 2004. 4, Culture and Society. Available at: https://www.ncbi.nlm.nih.gov/books/NBK216037/.

22. Jazieh AR, Volker S, Taher S. Involving the family in patient care: A culturally tailored communication model. Glob J Qual Saf Healthc 2018;1(2):33–7.

23. Shoemaker SJ, Wolf MS, Brach C. Development of the patient education materials assessment tool (PEMAT): A new measure of understandability and actionability for print and audiovisual patient information. Patient Educ Couns 2014;96(3):395–403.

24. Vishnevetsky J, Walters CB, Tan KS. Interrater reliability of the Patient Education Materials Assessment Tool (PEMAT). Patient Educ Couns 2018;101(3):490–6.

25. Grabeel KL, Russomanno J, Oelschlegel S, et al. Computerized versus hand-scored health literacy tools: A comparison of Simple Measure of Gobbledygook (SMOG) and Flesch-Kincaid in printed patient education materials. J Med Libr Assoc 2018;106(1):38–45.

26. Badarudeen S, Sabharwal S. Assessing readability of patient education materials: Current role in orthopaedics. Clin Orthop Rel Res 2010;468(10):2572–80.

27. Shneyderman M, Snow GE, Davis R, et al. Readability of online materials related to vocal cord leukoplakia. OTO Open 2021;5(3). 2473974X211032644. Published 2021 Aug 9.

28. Salmon C, O'Conor R, Sigh S, et al. Characteristics of outpatient clinical summaries in the United States. Int J Med Inf 2016;94:75–80.

29. Health Education Materials Assessment Tool. MedlinePlus. Available at: https://medlineplus.gov/pdf/health-education-materials-assessment-tool.pdf. [Accessed 11 December 2023].

30. Lecler A, Duron L, Soyer P. Revolutionizing radiology with GPT-based models: Current applications, future possibilities and limitations of chatgpt. Diagn Interv Imaging 2023;104(6):269–74.

31. U.S. National Library of Medicine. MedlinePlus. Available at: https://medlineplus.gov/. [Accessed 10 December 2023].

Patient Education on Genomics

Melissa Murfin, PharmD, BCACP, PA-C, DFAAPA

KEYWORDS

- Personalized medicine • Precision medicine • Genetic testing • Patient education
- Genetic counseling • Pharmacogenetics • Oncology • Prenatal genetic testing

KEY POINTS

- Genomics is a relatively new area of medicine with little direct guidance on patient education.
- Educating patients on genetic and genomic testing is multifaceted and may involve the patient as well as their family.
- Physician Assistants need skills in explaining the genetic science as well as empathy in assisting patients with processing implications of genetic test results.
- Patient education on genetic test results addresses ethical principles concerning privacy, confidentiality, patient autonomy, and storage and use of the patient's genetic material.
- Cultural humility assists with understanding that patients may decline to submit to genetic testing.

INTRODUCTION

Genomics is on the leading edge of medicine with applications across many disciplines, including primary care, psychiatry, pediatrics, reproductive health, and oncology. The idea of precision medicine, or personalized medicine, is of interest in clinical practice now that genetic and genomic testing is widely available with multiple uses in screening, diagnosis, and treatment of diseases. Understanding a patient's specific genetic variants can guide medication choices with pharmacogenetic testing or determination of cancer tumor markers. Prenatal genetic testing helps patients understand the potential risk of passing an inherited genetic condition to a fetus, prepare for the birth of a child with a genetic disorder, or consider the difficult decision of termination of a pregnancy. Genetic testing may also be diagnostic and help collate symptoms into a disease process that may be treated or better understood.

With the variety of genetic testing applications in medicine, it can be challenging for Physician Assistants (PAs) to provide appropriate patient education to assist patients

Physician Assistant Program, Ithaca College, School-Health-Sciences-and-Human-Performance, 953 Danby Road, Ithaca, NY 14850, USA
E-mail address: mmurfin@ithaca.edu

Physician Assist Clin 9 (2024) 601–614
https://doi.org/10.1016/j.cpha.2024.05.011
2405-7991/24/© 2024 Elsevier Inc.

in making decisions about their health based on genetic test results. From deciding whether to proceed with testing to understanding a diagnosis to making treatment decisions, the PA can be an important guide for their patients, who often must make life-altering decisions when faced with genetic test results. PAs possess the skills to distill the genetic science to a form patients can understand, explain the risk and benefit implications of proceeding with testing, and assist patients in making treatment decisions that align with the patient's values and beliefs.

OBJECTIVES

- Illustrate the history of genetics in medicine and the evolution of genetic and genomic testing.
- Compare and contrast different forms of genetic testing, including prenatal testing, oncology genetic testing, pharmacogenetic testing, diagnostic genetic testing, and direct-to-consumer genetic testing.
- Provide evidence-based recommendations on patient education on the different types of genetic testing.
- Recommend a systematic approach to patient education on genetic medicine with application to clinical practice.
- Use cultural humility when approaching patient education regarding genetic testing.

KEY CONCEPTS

- Genetics is the study of genes and how they are inherited. Genetic testing typically identifies variants in single genes.
- Genomics is the study of multiple genes and how the genes interact with each other and the environment. Genomic testing typically involves multiple genes in sequence.
- Genetic education and counseling help patients understand the risks and benefits of genetic testing to assist with making informed decisions on whether to undergo genetic testing and how to proceed with a medical management plan once results are available.[1]
- Prenatal genetic counseling may be completed before conception for patients with personal or family history of genetic disorders or after conception to screen for genetic disorders during a pregnancy.
- Oncology genetic testing may involve patient genetics or tumor genetics, both of which can be used to guide treatment.
- Pharmacogenetics is used in primary care, behavioral medicine, and pain management to determine genetic variants that affect the way the liver metabolizes drugs. These variants can lead to an increased likelihood of adverse effects or lack of efficacy.
- Direct-to-consumer testing involves testing that patients can elect without a laboratory order from their PA provider.

BACKGROUND AND CONTEXT
Historical Perspective

Genetics in medicine is a relatively new field that traces its beginnings to the latter half of the twentieth century.[2] Genetics was considered a basic research science with applications to anatomy and physiology, but not something understood or used in human medical practice. The term "human genetics" was not widely used until the late 1940s when the American Society of Human Genetics (ASHG) was formed and launched the American Journal of Human Genetics.[3] Further advances, such as the identification of the structure of DNA, advanced laboratory methods, and molecular technologies, led to the use of genetics in diagnostics, treatment, and patient counseling.[3]

Internal medicine physicians embraced genetics early with many moving into pediatrics and adapting genetics to the treatment of inherited childhood diseases.[4] Pediatric genetic conditions were termed "birth defects" and studied to determine if causality was associated with physical malformations at the genetic level, deformities that occurred because of external forces, or reversible defects related to external forces.[4] Inherited genetic conditions, such as Down syndrome, Turner syndrome, and Klinefelter syndrome, were identified in the late 1950s.[4] Other genetic conditions were referred to as inborn errors of metabolism and addressed through dietary changes.[3]

Genetic counseling and patient education were initially the role of the physician and incorporated into medical genetic clinic appointments.[4] Patients and their caregivers received information on the medical condition, risk of recurrence, and the implications (both medical and emotional) of a genetic disease in the family. A need to develop a profession of people who were specifically trained in genetic disease inheritance and patient and family support was identified. The genetic counseling profession was established at Sarah Lawrence College and graduated the first class of 8 genetic counselors in 1971.[4] The ASHG developed a formal definition of genetic counseling in 1975, which incorporated consideration of the burden of genetic disease on the affected family and the idea that specific communication techniques are needed to transmit this information to the family. At that time, genetic counseling involved explaining recessive genes and how genetic conditions are transmitted, risks associated with being a carrier, signs and symptoms of the condition, the possibilities of prenatal testing, and the potential necessity of testing other family members.[4]

Prenatal genetic screening to identify genetic disorders and identify sex of the fetus began in the 1950s when the first amniocentesis was performed.[5,6] Genetic malformations are the most common cause of fetal prenatal mortality and occur in approximately 1 in 150 live births.[5] Numerous diagnostic genetic testing methods are available for prenatal testing, including amniocentesis, chorionic villus sampling (CVS), and cordocentesis. These are all invasive processes that are relatively safe, however, still provide some risk to the fetus and mother. Screening was generally recommended only in high-risk pregnancies to offer options for diagnosis and treatment of genetic malformations or termination of pregnancy.[5]

CURRENT LANDSCAPE
Noninvasive Prenatal Genetic Testing

As genetic testing has improved, noninvasive methods for prenatal testing have been developed along with protocols for testing at specific times during pregnancy. Prenatal genetic screening has expanded from only screening high-risk pregnancies. In 2007, the American College of Obstetrics and Gynecology (ACOG) began offering recommended genetic testing for all pregnancies.[5] Prenatal genetic testing is now offered throughout pregnancy. First-trimester genetic screening involves ultrasound measurement of nuchal translucency for neural tube defects and serum testing for specific biochemical markers predictive of genetic disease, such as alpha human chorionic gonadotropin and other pregnancy-related proteins.[5]

The quadruple marker screening test or "Quad Screen" has been available since the 1990s and is performed in the 15th to 22nd weeks of pregnancy.[5] Contingent screening combines the first-trimester genetic screening with the quad screen. First-semester testing divides patients into high-, medium-, and low-risk groups. A high-risk patient is offered additional diagnostic testing, such as amniocentesis or CVS. Medium-risk patients proceed to the quad screen, whereas low-risk patients often need no additional testing.[5]

Noninvasive testing via cell-free DNA was developed in 2011 to offer safer options for prenatal screening for genetic abnormalities.[7] Cell-free DNA involves a blood test to collect fetal DNA that is circulating in the pregnant person's bloodstream. This testing can be performed as early as 10 weeks' gestation and detects sex of the fetus and conditions where an abnormal number of chromosomes are present, like Down syndrome and Turner syndrome.[7] Patient education during prenatal testing is complex owing to the implications of a positive genetic test on a current pregnancy, for future pregnancies, and for family members who may also be affected.

Oncology Genetic Testing

Genetic testing is used commonly in oncology to identify genetic variants or mutations that may be predictive of potential risk of developing inherited cancer. Patients who have been diagnosed with cancer may also undergo genetic testing to determine their risk of developing other cancers or if family members should also undergo genetic testing.[8] Genetic counselors are often involved in this process to discuss family history and the likelihood of family members developing cancers.

Another application of genetic testing in oncology is evaluating the presence or absence of specific markers on tumors that may guide treatment in breast cancer and other types of cancer. The oncology provider is an integral part of patient education in these cases, helping the patient to understand the test results and determine the best approach to treatment.[8]

Direct-to-Consumer Testing

In 2003, the Human Genome Project completed sequencing of more than 90% of the human genome.[9] Two years later, direct-to-consumer genetic testing companies began offering their products to consumers.[9] Now, access to personal genetic information has created a public interest in precision medicine with more than 26 million people participating in commercial genetic testing.[9] Lay people now have access to multiple types of genetic testing from determining potential ancestry links to disease risk profiles, which the patient can access directly without an order from a provider. This comes with some uncertainty, as the consumer is often left to determine interpretation of their own test results when patient education is not provided by the direct-to-consumer laboratories. Many consumers bring test results to their health care providers, who may not be prepared to interpret these results, which may include genetic variants that have little to no clinical significance.

Pharmacogenetic Testing

Pharmacogenetic testing was first performed in the 1950s but was thought to be lacking in utility until specific liver enzymes involved in drug metabolism were identified.[10] Testing is now available to determine genetic variants that affect a patient's ability to metabolize drugs, which assists the prescriber in predicting the potential for medication adverse effects or lack of efficacy. Additional genetic testing for markers associated with specific drugs can indicate whether medications should be contraindicated in affected patients because of the potential for life-threatening hypersensitivity reactions.

Clinical pharmacists are often tasked with the patient education of pharmacogenetic testing; however, PAs and other prescribers may use testing in clinical practice before prescribing a medication. The prescriber will need to educate the patient on the risks and benefits of getting the testing as well as counseling on the results.

THEORETIC FOUNDATIONS
Theoretic Frameworks

Many of the theoretic models of patient education on genomics come from the genetic counseling profession. Genetic counselors are trained to discuss the science behind the genetics, the medical implications of the test results, and the potential emotional impact of the test results on the patient and their family.[11] Genetic counselors approach this information delivery through a psychoeducational model that pairs psychotherapy techniques with patient education.[11] Specific techniques include the use of techniques also used in cognitive behavioral therapy and decision science.[12]

For PAs and other clinicians not specifically trained in genetic counseling, patient counseling models about informed consent and delivering bad news may be useful in discussing genetic testing results that involve life-altering diagnoses. Education on the informed consent process is important to assist patients in determining if the patient wishes to proceed with genetic testing and understands their test results. Patients must be made aware of potential ramifications of genetic testing for themselves and their family before electing to have any genetic testing performed. The use of empathy is vital when counseling patients on their results, as diagnostic testing may reveal life-altering genetic conditions.

Application to Patient Education

Patient education on genetic testing involves addressing the following:

- Informed consent for genetic testing
- The potential risk of inherited disease in the patient and family
- Diagnosis of genetic conditions
- Treatment of cancer
- Prognosis for disease treatment
- The variety of emotions a patient and their family may experience as they attempt to digest and process this complex information.

Decision science theory is useful to assist patients in determining whether to proceed with genetic testing and how to respond to the results. Medical decisions are based on science and best practice and include the patient's values and beliefs. This mirrors the theory that decisions are based on rational thought, which includes feelings, personality, and context.[12] Research about the concept of gain and loss indicates that most people are risk averse and will choose to avoid losing something of value rather than gaining something of equal value.[12] Framing decisions in terms of what the patient gains with genomic testing can be helpful when patients are attempting to make difficult decisions involving the treatment of an inherited condition.[12]

Fuzzy trace theory is also an application of decision science that is applicable to genomic patient education. Fuzzy trace theory indicates people will generally choose treatment that corresponds to what the essence of the condition is rather than the verbatim details.[12] For example, even when understanding details and statistics of cancer treatment, people tend to choose options based on a fuzzy perception of high or low risk or good or bad outcomes.[12]

Understanding how to proceed after a genetic disorder diagnosis may also represent a significant cognitive and emotional load for patients. Patients faced with decisions with an urgent timeline or that involve life-altering illness may make decisions guided by emotion rather than a complete understanding of all available options.[12] This may occur when parents are considering termination of pregnancy when a potentially fatal condition is revealed on prenatal fetal testing, as timing of the decision may be urgent and not allow for sufficient time to explore options that review risks and benefits of continuing the pregnancy.[12]

BEST PRACTICES AND STRATEGIES
Evidence-Based Approaches

Approaches a PA may use for patient education on genetic testing involve helping the patient understand the genetics of the condition, helping the patient understand the need for the genetic test, explaining the test results, and developing a plan for going forward, which may involve the patient and additional family members. Generally, evidence-based patient education must be patient-centered and offer significant patient engagement.[13] The Health Care Education Association guidelines recommend a systematic approach with 5 steps: Assessment, Planning, Education, Implementation, and Evaluation.[13] This process is as follows:

- Assessment of patient's learning needs
- Planning goal-setting strategies based on the learning needs assessment
- Choosing an appropriate educational model
- Focusing on the patient during implementation using active learning skills, concept reinforcement, and adjusting teaching as needed based on patient's understanding.
- Evaluation of patient's understanding with techniques like Teach Back and ultimately determining outcomes by measuring patient adherence with the proposed plan.[13]

The Teach Back method is an evidence-based approach commonly used by PAs in patient education to improve patient communication. The Teach Back method is an active learning technique and is useful in educating patients on genetic conditions as well. With the Teach Back method, the PA provides information to the patient, who is then asked to repeat what they heard for an assessment of their understanding.[14] This allows the PA to address any potential issues with health literacy by recognizing what the patient understood after patient counseling.

Many PAs are also trained in having difficult conversations, skills that can be translated to discussing genetic test results with patients. There are 3 specific patient counseling models used in difficult conversations that can be adapted to the discussion of genetic test results: Ask-Tell-Ask, SPIKES strategy, and the NURSE tool.[15]

The Ask-Tell-Ask method is a patient-centered, collaborative approach that involves asking open-ended questions to assess the patient's knowledge and emotional status before telling the patient the information that is needed about their genetic condition or test result, then asking again to determine the patient's understanding of the test results and/or treatment plan.[15]

The SPIKES protocol offers a stepwise approach to delivering difficult news that incorporates the Ask-Tell-Ask method.[15] The 6 steps of SPIKES are as follows:

1. Setup: creating an appropriate environment, both physical and emotional, for sharing potentially life-altering genetic information.

2. Perception: asking open-ended questions to establish the patient's perception of their medical condition.
3. Invitation: determining how much information the patient is ready to receive at the time of the conversation.
4. Knowledge: disclosing the information and checking for understanding.
5. Empathy: acknowledging and validating the patient's emotions as appropriate and expected for the situation.
6. Summary and strategy: determining the patient's readiness for discussing the next steps and developing the treatment plan.[15]

Empathy is an important part of genomics education, as patients may be dealing with complex feelings about diagnosis of an inherited disease or implications for family members or future pregnancies. The NURSE tool aids the PA in expressing empathy to the patient. The NURSE tool offers the following suggestions for empathetic responses:

- Naming the emotion the patient is experiencing
- Understanding and validating the emotion
- Respecting and acknowledging the emotional experience
- Supporting the patient as they process the information
- Exploring the patient's feelings by asking them to elaborate.[15]

Genomic patient education may be extended to additional family members who are undergoing testing and potential diagnosis of genetic illness. With prenatal testing, the parents may be faced with a decision to terminate a pregnancy or decide whether to attempt pregnancy owing to the risk of a child experiencing a traumatic illness. Genetic testing after a cancer diagnosis may guide treatment, which could offer hope for a positive outcome or suggest that treatment is likely to be unsuccessful and hospice or palliative care is indicated. Using a combination of educational techniques to ensure the patient understands the ramifications of the genetic condition and risks and benefits of treatment is critical to providing the utmost in patient care.

CASE STUDIES
Prenatal Testing Case

A US case that may be familiar involved a 31-year-old patient in Texas who received prenatal testing. The fetus was determined to have a genetic condition that was not compatible with life. Continuing the pregnancy was likely to harm the mother's health and possibly prevent her from future pregnancies. This diagnosis was devastating to the mother and her partner given the implications for the current pregnancy and those in the future. The case became a national story owing to legal issues around pregnancy termination.[16] Supporting the patient and their family through a case like this is difficult for any provider and could involve the use of empathy and the SPIKES protocol.

Cancer Genetics Case

A 57-year-old patient is diagnosed with breast cancer after routine mammography. Although her mother died in a car accident at age 42, she does recall an aunt who had breast cancer. The patient now faces 2 potential genetic tests: one to determine the characteristics of her tumor and guide treatment and one for the BRCA gene to determine the possibility of familial cancer. Counseling in this case could include the SPIKES protocol with Ask-Tell-Ask to determine what the patient knows about her cancer and what she would like to know, expressions of empathy, providing information to help her make treatment decisions, and assisting with the decision on whether and how to share this information with her family if the BRCA testing indicates a need for family testing.

Pharmacogenetics Case

A 28-year-old patient currently treated with paroxetine for major depressive disorder comes to clinic for follow-up. The patient notes no improvement of symptoms over the past 12 months of treatment. The PA elected to order pharmacogenomic testing, which included results for the metabolic liver enzymes, CYP2D6 and CYP2C19. The test indicated the patient had a genetic variant in CYP2D6 that would impair the efficacy of paroxetine and a normal metabolic pattern in CYP2C19. The PA consulted guidelines provided by the Clinical Pharmacogenetics Implementation Consortium (CPIC), which recommended choosing a drug other than paroxetine to treat the patient's depression.[17] In this case, Ask-Tell-Ask would be a helpful tool in gauging the patient's understanding of the genetic test, communicating the results, and determining the patient's perception of the implications on medication use.

PRACTICAL TIPS

A simple, structured approach to genomic education is beneficial for the patient and PA. Explaining what genetic testing does and the reasons for performing a genetic test are an effective way to start. The Centers for Disease Control and Prevention (CDC) recommends briefly explaining that genetic testing looks for a mutation or change in the DNA and that this can have implications for family members as well.[18] Possible reasons for genetic testing to communicate to a patient include the following:

- Identifying a potential disease before symptoms occur
- Diagnosing a genetic condition once symptoms are noted
- Determining the possibility of a genetic condition affecting a current or future pregnancy
- Guiding cancer treatment
- Determining how the patient may respond to certain medications.[18]

The Nebraska Department of Health and Human Services (DHHS) published an informed consent booklet with thorough guidance on education for patients before undergoing genomic testing.[19] The education process suggested by Nebraska DHHS includes explaining the following:

- Genetics and genetics tests
- The process of undergoing a genetic test
- What knowledge is gained from the genetic test and how that knowledge may be beneficial
- Limits and risks of genetic testing
- Possible test results and what results mean
- Options for treatment or moving forward with results
- Privacy considerations, including whether genetic material is stored or discarded
- Withdrawing consent.[19]

Cost of genetic testing is important to discuss with patients as part of the informed consent process. Genetic tests may not be covered by insurance, leading patients to decline genetic testing, which impacts access to care.

CHALLENGES AND CONSIDERATIONS
Existing Challenges: Cost

One of the biggest barriers associated with genetic testing is cost. Genetic testing can be hundreds or thousands of dollars in out-of-pocket medical expense and varies significantly according to the type and purpose of the genetic test. Prenatal testing is often the lowest cost and may be fully covered by insurance. Out-of-pocket costs may be less than $100.[20]

Genetic testing for cancers may be covered by private insurance and Medicare or Medicaid, depending on specifically defined parameters. The Centers for Medicaid and Medicare Services (CMS) has developed guidelines for coverage of some genetic tests.[20] Medicare will cover BRCA testing for patients with a personal history of breast cancer and specific indications, including age at diagnosis, family history of breast cancer in blood relatives, absence of breast cancer tumor markers, personal or family history of other cancers, or Ashkenazi Jewish descent.[20] Medicaid coverage varies by state with most states offering coverage, except Alabama.[21] Patients without insurance or who are underinsured may pay as much as $300 to $500 for BRCA testing.

In some cases, CMS will only cover genetic or genomic testing when the patient already has symptoms of cancer. For colon cancer owing to Lynch syndrome, Medicare typically will only cover testing in patients that are already experiencing symptoms.[21]

Pharmacogenetic testing has mixed insurance coverage with some private insurers increasing coverage over the past few years. Coverage for CYP2C19 testing to evaluate efficacy of clopidogrel (Plavix) is generally well established because of the efficacy data. Guidelines from CMS indicate there is coverage for some genetic tests related to medications based on recommendations from the Food and Drug Administration and CPIC.[22]

Existing Challenges: Provider Education

Another challenge includes the provider's familiarity with genetic testing and interpretation. The use of genetic testing varies across medical specialties and may not be something the PA has encountered in clinical practice or in great depth during PA training. One study indicated that genetics education is integrated into PA program curricula, however, is not standardized across programs and has limited contact hours, although medical genetic information has increased dramatically over the past decade.[23] PAs may be reluctant to order or provide genomic education to patients because of gaps in their own knowledge. Resources, like the Jackson Laboratory, are available to assist with improving provider knowledge of genetics and genomics.

ETHICAL CONSIDERATIONS

There are numerous potential ethical issues to consider when discussing genetic testing with patients. Conversations about confidentiality and storage and use of the patient's genetic material should be addressed during the informed consent process. The Genetic Information Nondiscrimination Act (GINA) took effect in 2009 and is federal protection for patients who undergo genetic testing.[24] The GINA prevents discrimination against employees based on personal or family genetic information and blocks medical insurers from using the results of genetic testing to determine insurance cost or eligibility.[24]

Addressing the storage and specific use of the patient's genetic material is an important part of the informed consent process. Questions may include where the genetic material samples are stored, for how long, and what the intended use is. The Havasupai Tribe in Arizona filed a lawsuit in 2004 against researchers at Arizona State University regarding the use of participants' DNA samples during research trials.[25] Tribal members elected to participate in a genetic study on type 2 diabetes and donated samples for that purpose. The participants later found that their genetic material had also been used in studies on schizophrenia and anthropologic research. As a result of the lawsuit, the study participants received their DNA samples, direct compensation, and indirect compensation in the form of money to be used for a clinic and school.[25] The informed consent process should clearly explain where the samples are being stored, how long before the samples will be discarded, and the intended use, particularly if there would be additional testing or research conducted on the samples.[22]

The basic ethical principle of patient autonomy also applies in patient education about genomics. Patients may make choices based on their preferences rather than clinical benefit. These types of decisions often occur when patients are faced with results of prenatal testing or cancer treatment.[11] Clinicians must recognize the ethical principle of patient autonomy in these situations and assist with implementation of a treatment plan that is consistent with the patient's beliefs and values.

Other issues include how to approach the results of testing. Direct-to-consumer tests may reveal unexpected family connections or a difference in paternity than what the patient understood. Laboratories that supply these tests may not have support structures in place to assist with adequate counseling on the ramifications of these results.[26] Legal opinion on whether genetic testing is reportable to family members who may also be affected has differed according to the case specifics.[26] Because of the delicacy of this information, PAs should include family member notification as a discussion point with the patient during the informed consent process to determine if the patient wishes to share test results with other family members.

CULTURAL AND DIVERSITY CONSIDERATIONS

Human genetics has a complicated history dating back to early identification of inherited disorders. The concept of eugenics developed with practices of eliminating individuals perceived to have unfavorable genetic conditions with the theory that these genetic conditions could be eliminated from the human gene pool.[3] Eugenics was a particular tenet of the Nazi holocaust and in states like North Carolina, a justification for forced sterilization of Black Americans in the twentieth century.[27] History of this nature may make it difficult for affected people to trust the idea of genetic testing and be willing to participate.

Cultural humility is important for all providers when exploring medical genetics. Recognizing diversity in beliefs and values includes consideration of beliefs about disease incidence and prevalence as well as appropriate treatment.[28] Some cultures may also have stigma associated with inherited conditions, as in the case with the Havasupai Tribe, who keep mental health conditions very private. These stigmas may lead patients to decline participation in genetic testing so as not to reveal an unwanted condition.[25] The Jackson Laboratory provides some guidance on how to increase culture competence in genetic medicine:

- Create a welcoming environment
- Use equitable collection of personal and family history
- Use interpreter services
- Use implicit bias training
- Increase diversity in the genomic workforce.[28]

FUTURE DIRECTIONS AND OPPORTUNITIES
Emerging Trends

Research into cost-effectiveness of genetic testing has the potential to improve implementation and insurance coverage. A recent study from Canada showed that implementation of pharmacogenomic testing before antidepressant prescription could save one province nearly $5000 per patient.[29] A study in the United States showed that genomic screening for Lynch syndrome as a predictor of colorectal cancer could improve quality-adjusted life-years.[30] Additional data involving implementation of genetic testing before prescribing could potentially improve patient outcomes. This could lead to greater engagement and demand for genomic patient education by providers.

RESOURCES

- General information on genetics and genomics
  - Society for PAs in Genetics and Genomics (SPAGG) https://spagg.wildapricot.org/
  - National Human Genome Research Institute (NHGRI) https://www.genome.gov/
  - CDC Public Health Genomics and Precision Health Knowledge Base https://phgkb.cdc.gov/PHGKB/phgHome.action?action=home
  - The Jackson Laboratory https://www.jax.org/
- Cancer Genetics Risk Assessment and Counseling https://www.cancer.gov/about-cancer/causes-prevention/genetics/risk-assessment-pdq
- ACOG Prenatal Genetic Testing Chart. https://www.acog.org/womens-health/infographics/prenatal-genetic-testing-chart
- Pharmacogenetics
  - Clinical Pharmacogenetics Implementation Consortium (CPIC) https://cpicpgx.org/
  - PharmGKB https://www.pharmgkb.org/
  - CMS Billing and Coding: Pharmacogenomics Testing https://www.cms.gov/medicare-coverage-database/view/article.aspx?articleid=58801&ver=40&

RECOMMENDATIONS

Recommendations for future practice in medical genetics include improving access to care, decreasing costs and improving insurance coverage of genetic testing, increasing implementation, and expanding provider education on ordering and interpreting genetic tests.

SUMMARY

Genomic medicine is part of many medical specialties and will continue to evolve with better testing techniques and understanding of the implications of genetic test results. The increasing use of genetics in medicine has led to a significant need for genetics professionals,[31] which offers opportunities for PAs to excel in this specialty. PAs have an important role in genomic education for patients and can help with understanding when to order genetic testing, the potential risks and benefits, and how to approach the results. Empathy and cultural humility are important parts of the genomic education process owing to significant ethical considerations about the use of a patient's genetic material.

KEY TAKEAWAYS

- Patient genomic education is complex and may include screening, diagnostic, and treatment testing.
- PAs can fill an important gap in medical genetics and provide patient education in genomic testing.
- Counseling patients on genetic tests can involve assisting patients in making serious, life-altering decisions.
- Patient education models that can be applied to patient genomic education include the Teach Back method, Ask-Tell-Ask, and the SPIKES protocol.
- Empathy and cultural humility are important components of patient education about genetic testing. The PA should be sensitive to historic abuses of power about genetics and cultural mores that may affect patients' willingness to undergo genetic testing.
- Cost of genetic testing continues to be a barrier to access to genetic testing for patients who are uninsured or underinsured.

CLINICS CARE POINTS

- PAs can play an important role in genetics education for patients.
- Check patient out-of-pocket costs before ordering genetic testing.
- Understand the implications of genetic testing for the individual patient.
- Recognize informed consent and issues with disclosure of genetic test results to family members.
- Recognize diversity and cultural barriers to genetic testing.

DISCLOSURE

The author has nothing to disclose.

REFERENCES

1. Cancer Genetics Risk Assessment and Counseling (PDQ) – Health Professional Version. National Cancer Institute. Available at: https://www.cancer.gov/about-cancer/causes-prevention/genetics/risk-assessment-pdq. [Accessed 15 January 2024].
2. Passarge E. Origins of human genetics. A personal perspective. Eur J Hum Genet 2021;29:1038–44.
3. Rimoin D, Hirschhorn K. A History of Medical Genetics in Pediatrics. Pediatr Res 2004;56:150–9.
4. Corson BL, Bernhardt BA. The evolution of genetic counseling at Johns Hopkins Hospital and beyond. Am J Med Genet 2021;185A:3230–5.
5. Carlson LM, Vora NL. Prenatal Diagnosis: Screening and Diagnostic Tools. Obstet Gynecol Clin North Am 2017;44(2):245–56.
6. Jindal A, Sharma M, Karena ZV, et al. Amniocentesis. In: StatPearls [Internet]. Treasure Island (FL): StatPearls Publishing; 2023. Available at: https://www.ncbi.nlm.nih.gov/books/NBK559247/.
7. Mahdi Mortazavipour M, Mahdian R, Shahbazi S. The current applications of cell-free fetal DNA in prenatal diagnosis of single-gene diseases: A review. Int J Reprod Biomed 2022;20(8):613–26. Published 2022 Sep 6.

8. Understanding Genetic Testing for Cancer Risk. American Cancer Society. Available at: https://www.cancer.org/cancer/risk-prevention/genetics/genetic-testing-for-cancer-risk/understanding-genetic-testing-for-cancer.html. [Accessed 13 January 2024].

9. Direct-to-Consumer Genetic Testing FAQ For Healthcare Professionals. National Human Genome Research Institute. Available at: https://www.genome.gov/For-Health-Professionals/Provider-Genomics-Education-Resources/Healthcare-Provider-Direct-to-Consumer-Genetic-Testing-FAQ#:~:text=Direct%2Dto%2Dconsumer%20genetic%20tests,risks)%20from%20a%20saliva%20sample&. [Accessed 16 April 2024].

10. Somogy A. Evolution of pharmacogenomics. Proc West Pharmacol Soc 2008; 51:1–4.

11. Biesecker B. Genetic Counseling and the Central Tenets of Practice. Cold Spring Harb Perspect Med 2020;10(3):a038968. Published 2020 Mar 2.

12. Biesecker B, Austin J, Caleshu C. Theories for Psychotherapeutic Genetic Counseling: Fuzzy Trace Theory and Cognitive Behavior Theory. J Genet Couns 2017; 26(2):322–30.

13. Cutilli C, Christensen S, Aloupis M, et al. Patient Education Practice Guidelines for Healthcare Professionals. Health Care Education Association. Available at: https://www.hcea-info.org/assets/hcea%20guidelines_BW%201-25-2021.pdf. (Accessed 16 April 2024).

14. Johnson JL, Moser L, Garwood CL. Health literacy: a primer for pharmacists. Am J Health Syst Pharm 2013;70(11):949–55.

15. Svarovsky T. Having Difficult Conversations: The Advanced Practitioner's Role. J Adv Pract Oncol 2013;4(1):47–52.

16. Klibanoff E. Kate Cox's case reveals how far Texas intends to go to enforce abortion laws. The Texas Tribune 2023. Available at: https://www.texastribune.org/2023/12/13/texas-abortion-lawsuit/. [Accessed 16 January 2024].

17. Bousman CA, Stevenson JM, Ramsey LB, et al. Clinical Pharmacogenetics Implementation Consortium (CPIC) Guideline for CYP2D6, CYP2C19, CYP2B6, SLC6A4, AND HTR2A Genotypes and Serotonin Reuptake Inhibitor Antidepressants. Clin Pharmacol Ther 2023;114(1):51–8.

18. Genetic testing. centers for disease control and prevention. Available at: https://www.cdc.gov/genomics/gtesting/genetic_testing.htm. [Accessed 15 January 2024].

19. Institute of Medicine (US) Committee on Assessing Genetic Risks. In: Andrews LB, Fullarton JE, Holtzman NA, et al, editors. Assessing genetic risks: implications for health and social policy. Washington (DC): National Academies Press (US); 1994. 7, Financing of Genetic Testing and Screening Services. Available at: https://www.ncbi.nlm.nih.gov/books/NBK236036/.

20. Local Coverage Determination (LCD). BRCA1 and BRCA2 Genetic Testing. Centers for Medicare and Medicaid Services. Available at: https://www.cms.gov/medicare-coverage-database/view/lcd.aspx?lcdId=36499&ver=24. [Accessed 15 January 2024].

21. Alabama. genetics policy hub. 2023. Available at: https://geneticspolicy.nccrcg.org/medicaid-policy/alabama/. [Accessed 15 January 2024].

22. Local Coverage Determination (LCD). MolDX: pharmacogenomics testing. Available at: https://www.cms.gov/medicare-coverage-database/view/lcd.aspx?lcdid=38294&ver=19. [Accessed 16 January 2024].

23. Patterson WG, Tribble LM, Hopkins CS, et al. The State of Genetics and Genomics Education in US Physician Assistant Programs. J Physician Assist Educ 2023;34(3):195–202.
24. Genetic information. U.S. Department of Health and Human Services. Available at: https://www.hhs.gov/hipaa/for-professionals/special-topics/genetic-information/index.html. [Accessed 16 January 2024].
25. Garrison NA. Genomic Justice for Native Americans: Impact of the Havasupai Case on Genetic Research. Sci Technol Human Values 2013;38(2):201–23.
26. Ethical Issues in Genetic Testing. The American College of Obstetricians and Gynecologists. 2020. Available at: https://www.acog.org/clinical/clinical-guidance/committee-opinion/articles/2008/06/ethical-issues-in-genetic-testing. [Accessed 16 January 2024].
27. Kickler TL. Eugenics board. North Carolina history Project. 2016. Available at: https://northcarolinahistory.org/encyclopedia/eugenics-board/. [Accessed 16 January 2024].
28. Steinmark L. Practicing culturally competent genomic medicine. The Jackson Laboratory; 2021. Available at: https://www.jax.org/news-and-insights/jax-blog/2021/december/practicing-culturally-competent-genomic-medicine. [Accessed 16 January 2024].
29. Ghanbarian S, Wong GWK, Bunka M, et al. Cost-effectiveness of pharmacogenomic-guided treatment for major depression. CMAJ 2023;195(44): E1499–508.
30. Guzauskas GF, Jiang S, Garbett S, et al. Cost-effectiveness of population-wide genomic screening for Lynch Syndrome in the United States. Genet Med 2022; 24(5):1017–26.
31. Raspa M, Moultrie R, Toth D, et al. Barriers and facilitators to genetic service delivery models: scoping review. Interact J Med Res 2021;10(1):e23523. Published 2021 Feb 25.

The Economics of Health Education

Trisha Harris, DHA, MS, PA-C[a],*, Laura Okolie, DMSc, MBA, MHS, PA-C[b]

KEYWORDS

- Health education • Economic policy • Billing • Coding • Reimbursement

KEY POINTS

- Despite advancements in health care delivery services, patient education continues to lag behind in the health system leading to poor outcomes.
- Patient education plays a pivotal role in reducing health care costs and in achieving improved health outcomes.
- Effective health education can improve patient safety and reduce readmissions.
- Comprehensive understanding of the connection between patient education and health care economics is essential.

INTRODUCTION

In the modern era of health care, patient education has transcended its traditional role as a simple information exchange. It has evolved into a critical factor in enhancing patient outcomes and shaping the economics of health care systems.[1] The promotion of health through education entails both costs and benefits. This study conducts a thorough exploration of "The Economics of Health Education," with a specific focus on billing for patient education, coding practices, group education, and the substantial savings that can be achieved through the prevention of hospital readmissions.

Crucially, this study also examines the theoretic foundations that underpin patient education strategies and their direct impact on the economics of health care. Understanding these theoretic models—such as the health belief model (HBM), theory of planned behavior (TPB), social cognitive theory (SCT), and the transtheoretical model (TTM)—is essential for designing effective patient education that can lead to significant economic benefits. These models provide the scaffolding for tailoring education to patient needs, thereby optimizing economic outcomes in health care delivery.

[a] University of Maryland Eastern Shore, 30665 Student Services Center, Princess Anne, MD 21853, USA; [b] Duke University School of Medicine, 800 South Duke Street, Box 104780, Durham, NC 27701, USA
* Corresponding author.
E-mail address: trishaharrispac@gmail.com

Physician Assist Clin 9 (2024) 615–631
https://doi.org/10.1016/j.cpha.2024.06.003
physicianassistant.theclinics.com
2405-7991/24/© 2024 Elsevier Inc. All rights are reserved, including those for text and data mining, AI training, and similar technologies.

Overview

The health care landscape in the twenty-first century is undergoing profound transformations, marked by extraordinary technological advances, evolving health care models, and shifting paradigms in patient care. Amid these changes, patient education has gained central importance, extending well beyond the mere dissemination of knowledge to individuals seeking care. It is increasingly recognized as an essential instrument for improving health outcomes, enhancing patient satisfaction, and notably, influencing the economics of health care delivery.[1]

Objectives

The primary objective of this study is to discuss the intricate relationship between patient education and health care economies. This includes exploration of the following key aspects:

- *Billing for patient education:* In this section, an examination is conducted to understand how patient education can be billed and reimbursed effectively within the modern health care system. The focus is on illuminating the financial mechanisms that facilitate its recognition as a reimbursable service.
- *Coding:* This study delves into the intricacies of coding for patient education, offering insights into the processes and frameworks facilitating the translation of educational efforts into tangible financial transactions.
- *Group education:* The concept of group education in health care is scrutinized, emphasizing its potential for imparting knowledge to a larger audience while offering unique economic advantages.
- *Savings by increased efficiencies*: One of the most compelling aspects of patient education in the context of health care economics is the potential for increased efficiencies within health care systems, such as reduced hospital readmission rates. Specifically, it examines how patient education interventions can mitigate the financial burden of recurrent hospital stays, benefiting both health care institutions and patients. This highlights the economic value of investing in patient education, underscoring its role in enhancing overall health care cost-efficiency.

Key Concepts and Definitions

To establish the foundation of our discussion, it is essential to introduce key concepts.

- *Patient education*: This term encompasses a spectrum of activities and interventions designed to empower patients with knowledge, skills, and confidence to actively participate in their own health care.[1]
- *Billing for education*: Billing for patient education refers to the process of documenting and seeking reimbursement for educational services provided to patients, either individually or in group settings.
- *Coding:* In the context of patient education, coding involves translating the educational content and delivery into standardized codes that facilitate billing and reimbursement.
- *Group education:* Group education in health care involves delivering educational content to multiple patients simultaneously, offering potential efficiency and cost-saving advantages.
- *Savings by increased efficiencies:* Effective patient education can lead to increased efficiencies within health care systems, notably through reduced hospital readmission rates. This not only diminishes the financial burden on health

care institutions but also benefits patients by decreasing the frequency of stressful and costly hospital stays.[2]

In the upcoming sections, the exploration of the economics of health education unfolds. This journey encompasses the historical evolution of patient education, its current landscape, and the theoretic foundations that underpin it. Furthermore, evidence-based best practices, a case study, and practical guidance for health care professionals and educators are presented.

Despite the challenges, which include barriers and ethical dilemmas, the exploration delves into the influence of cultural and diversity considerations on patient education. The investigation extends into the future, identifying emerging trends in digital tools and resources that hold the promise of reshaping the economic impact of patient education.

Concluding the study, the summary of key takeaways emphasizes the pivotal role of patient education in achieving improved health outcomes and cost-effective health care. The ultimate objective is to provide a comprehensive understanding of the connection between patient education and health care economics, with the aim of fostering a patient-centered health care system.

BACKGROUND AND CONTEXT

Health education is essential in every aspect of successful health care delivery. It is important to recognize the levels of complexity involved with health education secondary to the complexity of disease processes. According to the National Center for Chronic Disease Prevention and Health Promotion, of the US$4.1 trillion spent on annual health care, 90% is allocated to individuals with chronic disease and mental health conditions.[3] Heart disease and stroke are the number one cause of death in the United States resulting in a cost of over US$216 billion per year to the health care system and US$147 billion secondary to loss of job productivity.[3] Annually, 1.7 million people are diagnosed with cancer, and over 600,000 people succumb to the disease making it the second leading cause of death in the United States. Economically, the medical care associated with the diagnosis and treatment of cancer continues to rise and is expected to reach more than US$240 billion by 2030.[3] Over 37 million people in the United States have type 2 diabetes. More than twice as many are at risk of developing the disease. The complications associated with type 2 diabetes such as blindness, diabetic nephropathy, diabetic neuropathy, amputations, and bacterial or fungal infection can surmount to cost over US$300 billion a year. The prevention of diseases such as to heart disease, stroke and diabetes, begins with examining the obesity epidemic in the United States.

The delivery of effective health education begins with the medical training of health care professionals to understand and apply evidence-based medicine to health care practices.[4] Health education involves a continuous realm of advancements in medicine, research, and technology that makes its possibilities infinite. Ideally, the end results surmount to patients and communities that receive long-term health benefits while providers and health care systems maintain some type of economic stability to continue to provide quality, affordable, and accessible health care for the communities in which they serve.

Historical Perspective

Health education has evolved from a provider-led communication to a platform focused on patient-centered care and shared decision-making.[2] The challenge arises in how to account for this transition in health education that result in economic stability. Previous studies have revealed that individuals were able to effectively improve their health through behavioral modification from acquired skills and patient education.[1,2] The new concept of health education that evolved focused on patient accountability for their own health outcomes without necessarily accounting for health inequalities secondary to low health literacy or social determinants of health (SDoHs).[1,5]

It can no longer be ignored that communities disproportionately affected by low-income and low health literacy result in health inequalities.[5,6] Health inequalities perpetuate poor health economics because it fails to establish the relationship between social inequalities with SDoHs. Health education may be the most important determining factor that eliminates health inequalities while perpetuating improved health outcomes and health economics.[1,5]

Stages in the development of patient education

Culturally influenced societal changes, disease morbidity, and mortality are all contributing factors in the development stages of health education and economics.[7] Geographic location, socioeconomic status (SES), and education are also contributing factors of evolution in health education and economics.[5,8] Economic benefits were nonexistent in the early stages in the development of patient education. The focus was to prevent the spread of diseases that could ultimately lead to death. In addition, the power of patient education and autonomy to "healthy self" was not yet grasped.[1,2]

The need for health education in hospitals became apparent through readmissions due to a lack of understanding of disease process, medication management, and chronic diseases.[9,10] Again, the benefits of educating health care professionals and patients were evident but the mechanism remained ambiguous.[4] The financial gain from preventing hospital readmissions as well as the associated liability for the institution would clearly be an economic benefit. The paradigm shift of placing a price tag on the educational aspect of health care is not a new concept, but to date, processes to support financial gain have not been implemented to its full potential within the health care industry.[7,8]

Current Landscape

The utilization of health education for health promotion and disease prevention is necessary for effective health care delivery. However, the mechanism of how health education is linked to the financial benefits has continued to evolve over the last several decades. According to Nutbeam, the terms health education and health literacy are mutually inclusive and often used interchangeably.[6] An assessment of health literacy should be performed to assess the impact of the health education delivery.[5,9] The evolution of social media allows access to a substantial amount of health information. This form of group education involves the mass delivery of information to individuals within a short period. Although efficient in its delivery to large populations simultaneously, this mechanism of group education also presents challenges in the oversight of the quality and the reliability of information delivered.[5,6] The coronavirus disease 2019 pandemic is an example of the use of social media for group education that ultimately impacted the perception of disease and treatment choices by the general public.

The economics of group health education and its long-term health and financial benefits are not clearly defined in the literature but is predicted to have a positive correlation in health promotion and intervention strategies, especially in populations that are considered medically underrepresented.[5,7] Equity, must also be considered in the economics of health education since studies show there are apparent disparities in health care strongly linked to health literacy and SES.[5,7,8]

THEORETIC FOUNDATIONS

In the realm of health care, patient education serves as a critical bridge between health care providers and their patients, aiming to empower individuals with the knowledge and skills necessary to manage their health effectively. While the importance of patient education in improving health outcomes is widely recognized, understanding the theoretic foundations that underpin patient education and its financial implications is equally essential. In this section, we delve into the theoretic frameworks that provide the theoretic scaffolding for patient education and how these frameworks can be practically applied within the context of patient education with a focus on its financial aspects.

Theoretic Frameworks Underpinning Patient Education

Patient education is not a one-size-fits-all practice; rather, it is rooted in various theoretic frameworks and models that guide its design and implementation. These theoretic underpinnings help health care professionals tailor patient education interventions to the unique needs and circumstances of individual patients.

Health belief model

The HBM is a well-established framework in health care that posits that an individual's health-related behavior is influenced by their perceptions of the severity of a health issue, their susceptibility to it, the benefits of taking preventive actions, and the barriers to doing so.[2] In patient education, HBM helps identify the key factors that shape a patient's willingness to engage in self-care activities. Health care providers can use this model to assess a patient's perceived barriers to accessing education, implementing treatment recommendations and design interventions to address these barriers.

Theory of planned behavior

TPB asserts that a person's intentions to engage in a behavior are determined by their attitudes, outcome expectations, self-efficacy, and perceived results due to adherence.[2] In the context of patient education, TPB is instrumental in understanding the factors that influence a patient's willingness to participate actively in their health care. By addressing patient attitudes and subjective norms, health care providers can shape educational interventions that align with a patient's intentions.

Social cognitive theory

SCT emphasizes the role of observational learning and self-regulation in behavior change.[11] In patient education, SCT can guide the development of educational programs that focus on modeling and reinforcement. Patients can learn from observing others' health behaviors, and they can develop self-efficacy in managing their health conditions. By incorporating SCT, patient education can foster self-efficacy and self-regulation in patients.

Transtheoretical model

TTM is a stages-of-change model that recognizes that individuals go through different stages when adopting new behaviors. These stages include precontemplation, contemplation, preparation, action, and maintenance.[2] In patient education, this model can help health care providers tailor their educational interventions to the patient's specific stage of readiness for change. This personalized approach can enhance the effectiveness of patient education.

Application of Theoretic Frameworks in Patient Education

Understanding the theoretic foundations is only the beginning. The true value of these frameworks lies in their practical application within patient education. By employing these models effectively, physician assistants (PAs) can enhance the impact of their patient education efforts, both in terms of health outcomes and financial implications.

Application of health belief model

In practice, HBM can guide health care professionals in assessing patients' perceived barriers to accessing patient education. For example, if a patient is apprehensive about attending educational sessions due to logistical or financial challenges, health care providers can address these concerns by offering alternative formats (eg, online education) or providing information on available financial assistance programs.

Application of theory of planned behavior

TPB can be practically applied by understanding a patient's attitudes, subjective norms, and perceived behavioral control in relation to their health care. Health care providers can customize patient education materials and interventions to align with a patient's beliefs and intentions. For example, if a patient holds negative attitudes toward medication adherence, interventions can focus on changing these attitudes through education and support. This is imperative because research indicates that increased adherence to disease-modifying therapies or medications can effectively slow down disease progression, ultimately leading to reduced health care resource utilization and associated costs.[12]

Application of social cognitive theory

SCT can be integrated into patient education by using role models and peer support to encourage behavior change. In a group education setting, for instance, health care providers can incorporate success stories from patients who have effectively managed their health conditions. Additionally, SCT principles can be employed to enhance self-efficacy by providing patients with the tools and skills needed for self-regulation.

Application of transtheoretical model

TTM's stages of change can be practically applied by tailoring interventions to a patient's readiness for change. For example, a patient in the precontemplation stage may require different support and education than a patient in the action stage. Understanding a patient's stage of change (**Table 1**) allows health care providers to offer the most relevant and effective patient education.[13]

These theoretic frameworks offer health care professionals valuable tools for designing and implementing patient education programs that are not only evidence-based but also customized to the unique needs and situations of patients. In doing so, health care professionals enhance patient outcomes and simultaneously contribute to the financial sustainability of health care systems by reducing unnecessary resource utilization and hospital readmissions. As the exploration of the economic aspects of patient education continues, it becomes evident that the application of these theories amplifies the efficiency and effectiveness of educational interventions, ultimately benefiting both patients and the health care system as a whole.

BEST PRACTICES AND STRATEGIES
Health and Financial Literacy

First, to provide effective and efficient care that are economically beneficial and sustainable, the provider must first understand the intricacies of reimbursements. Second, reducing error in billing, coding, and documentation reduces the providers' risk of fraud and abuse allegations.[14] This includes adherence to requirements set forth

Table 1 Guide for clinical practice		
Stages of Change	**Patient Characteristics**	**Provider Strategies**
Precontemplation	Denial and deflection. Argumentative	Express concern. Ask permission to discuss and identify discrepancies. Provide information
Contemplation	Open to discussion and understand the need for change. Can be obsessive but ready to commit to goals	Elicit patients' perspective, pros and cons, and suggest trials. Provide resources for support
Preparation and determination	Procrastination but can overcome obstacles. Able to follow a plan	Set start date. Formal agreement/contract. Publicly announce and recruit support system. Slip vs relapse
Action	Committed but vulnerable. Focused action plan. Struggle with long-term goals	Reassess, readjust, and re-emphasize plan and expectations
Maintenance	Wavering commitment. Lifestyle that supports change	Reduce risk of relapse. Reflect on long-term goals rather than short-term gratification

Note: From Feldman MD, Christensen JF, eds. *Behavioral Medicine: A Guide for clinical Practice*, 4th ed. New York: McGraw-Hill Education; 2014.

by federal, state, and private insurance payers, knowledge of the provider fee schedule, and reimbursement rates.[14,15] In addition, one must understand what services are covered by the patient's health care plan and how much the payer is willing to reimburse for services provided. Failing to understand the above will lead to unnecessary out-of-pocket cost for the patient and lack of coverage for patient education performed by the provider. It is, therefore, imperative that health care providers become knowledgeable about health care systems including insurance reimbursements and plan coverages. Strengthening the health and financial literacy of the health care provider allows them to pass along this knowledge to their patients and the two can work together to obtain the best care for the patient.

Medicare, Medicaid, and Private Insurance

Medical treatments and interventions are not always evidence-based. Patient care is not always outcome-driven, and therefore, prevention is not always at the forefront of patient care. Financial incentives serves as one way to alter the behavior of health care providers that ultimately benefit patient outcomes.[14] Outcome-driven and evidence-based medicine must be standardized to support best practices in the delivery of patient care. The Center for Medicare and Medicaid Services (CMS) historically sets the health care delivery and reimbursement standards for federal, government, and private payers.[15] Following these standards brings financial incentives for providers and health benefits for patients. Pay for performance and value-based reimbursements are examples of 2 incentive programs in which both patient and provider benefit if implemented appropriately. More importantly, standardization should allow for measurable outcome based on quality of care objectives and reassessment to allow for adjustments and improvement in patient outcomes. Incentives must be given to support long-term goals and outcomes, not just for completing particular task such as office, procedures, and documentation.[14] Violating these standards, however, can result in penalties, fees, and legal repercussions for the provider and the institution where any infractions may have occurred. Private insurance companies commonly follow the standards set forth by CMS. Patient deductibles, copays, and provider reimbursements are dependent upon the type of plan for which the patient receives coverage and whether the provider is considered in-network or out-of-network.

Provider Reimbursements: Fee Schedule, Fee for Service, and Value-based Reimbursements

It behooves providers to understand the associated fee schedule for patient education for billing purposes. The difference between what is billed to a payer, what is written off by the provider, and the financial responsibility of the patient, all rely on the approved Medicare fee schedule.[15] Providers must also recognize that the amount billed for services does not necessarily equate to what will be reimbursed.[14] Case 13.1 gives an example of a patient scenario in which the provider must write off what is neither considered reimbursable by the payer nor deemed the financial responsibility of the patient. Write-offs result in a loss of perceived income to the practice for services provided.

Health care reform has attempted to move away from fee for service reimbursements, which often supports high patient volumes and uncoordinated care with little regard for quality of care and patient outcomes. Value-based reimbursement, however, supports the economic benefits in health education. Medicare has already adopted similar pay for performance initiatives to decrease health care disparities and improve the quality of care.[16]

CHALLENGES AND CONSIDERATIONS

In the health care domain, patient education, acknowledged for its pivotal contribution to enhancing health care outcomes, is characterized by a multifaceted interplay of economic challenges, ethical dilemmas, and cultural factors. Within this section, a thorough exploration is conducted to unravel the complexities of challenges and economic aspects inherent with patient education, with a primary emphasis on its financial consequences and its influence on the broader landscape of health care economics.

Existing Challenges in Patient Education

Effective billing

The health care system's billing practices are inherently complex and multifaceted. Billing for patient education is no exception to this complexity. One major challenge is the varying reimbursement policies across different health care settings and payers. A lack of standardized billing codes and procedures can hinder health care professionals from accurately and consistently billing for patient education services. Inconsistent documentation and coding practices can lead to lost revenue and hinder the financial sustainability of patient education programs.

Adding to these challenges, the landscape of reimbursement is frequently updated, necessitating continuous education and vigilant monitoring to stay current with the latest billing requirements. These changes can significantly impact how patient education services are billed and reimbursed. Without an ongoing commitment to education and adaptation, health care providers may find it increasingly difficult to secure appropriate reimbursement, compounding financial challenges and affecting the viability of patient education initiatives.

Accurate coding
The coding of patient education encounters presents another challenge. Assigning appropriate ICD-10 codes for educational services provided to patients is crucial not only for billing but also for tracking and evaluating the effectiveness of educational interventions. However, coding errors can occur, leading to underreporting of educational services and potentially affecting reimbursement. Ensuring accurate coding is essential to reflect the true scope of patient education efforts.

Group education
Group education programs offer numerous advantages, including cost-effectiveness and the potential for shared learning experiences. Nevertheless, they come with their own set of challenges. Patient heterogeneity in a group setting necessitates tailoring education to meet individual needs within the group. Balancing personalized education with the efficiency of group sessions can be challenging. Furthermore, logistical issues, such as scheduling, coordinating participants, and securing appropriate facilities, can pose significant obstacles to the successful implementation of group education.

Ethical Considerations in the Economics of Patient Education

Ethical dilemmas are intricately interwoven with the economic aspects of patient education:

Financial incentives versus patient welfare
Balancing financial incentives with patient welfare is an ethical tightrope. PAs, other members of the health care team and institutions may face pressures to maximize billable educational services for financial gain. This dynamic raises ethical concerns regarding the primary motivation behind patient education. Striking the right balance between financial considerations and genuine patient well-being is an ongoing ethical challenge.

Patient autonomy and informed consent
Respecting patient autonomy and obtaining informed consent are fundamental ethical principles. In the context of patient education, this involves ensuring that patients understand the financial aspects of the education provided and the potential costs involved. Patients should be fully informed about the potential costs and financial implications, upholding ethical standards and autonomy.

Privacy and data security
As patient education increasingly incorporates digital tools, the ethical imperative of data privacy and security becomes paramount. Protecting patient information and ensuring compliance with privacy regulations are not only ethical imperatives but also economic considerations. Breaches in data security can have profound financial implications and erode patient trust.

Cultural and Diversity Considerations in the Economics of Patient Education

Cultural and diversity factors introduce a unique dimension to the economic landscape of patient education:

Language and communication
Language barriers can significantly impact the economics of patient education. Ensuring accessible and comprehensible educational materials and sessions for diverse linguistic backgrounds may require translation services, multilingual

resources, and culturally sensitive communication. This addresses an economic challenge while maintaining cultural inclusivity.

Cultural beliefs and health literacy

Cultural beliefs and diverse levels of health literacy play a significant role in shaping the effectiveness of patient education, thereby influencing its economic implications. Understanding and acknowledging cultural differences in health care practices are essential components of delivering education that is culturally sensitive and effective.

Furthermore, it is important to recognize that health literacy is acknowledged as a key SDoH outcome. Individuals with higher levels of health literacy are more likely to actively engage in preventive behaviors, make informed health care decisions, and effectively manage their health conditions.[1,17] This, in turn, can result in improved health outcomes and a reduction in costly interventions. Thus, the economic impact of patient education is intricately linked to cultural considerations and health literacy levels, underscoring the importance of addressing these factors in the pursuit of cost-effective health care and favorable patient outcomes.

Health disparities and socioeconomic factors

Socioeconomic factors and health disparities are inherently connected to the economic challenges faced by health care systems. Addressing these disparities is crucial from both ethical and economic standpoints. The reduction of health inequities holds the potential to alleviate the overall economic strain on health care systems, fostering financial sustainability.

Patient education emerges as a valuable tool in this endeavor, as it has the potential to mitigate health care disparities and enhance health equity.[18] Limited health literacy often contributes to disparities in patient-reported outcomes.[18] However, by offering education that is both accessible and tailored to diverse populations, health care systems empower patients to take an active role in their health care. This, in turn, leads to improved health outcomes and a reduction in disparities. Therefore, the economic impact of patient education is intrinsically linked to addressing cultural and diversity considerations and achieving greater equity in health care, ultimately benefiting both patients and the health care system.

Educating patients about the significance of regular and preventive care, including the role of a primary care provider or medical home, can substantially mitigate nonurgent emergency service use. This approach alleviates system strain and reduces costs related to unnecessary procedures and tests. Importantly, focusing on these educational aspects can also address health disparities and socioeconomic factors. By ensuring all patients, regardless of background or economic status, understand how to access and utilize preventive care effectively, health care systems can enhance health equity and reduce disparities in health care access. This not only improves health outcomes but also contributes to the overall cost-efficiency of the health care system, demonstrating a crucial linkage among patient education, health equity, and economic savings.[19]

Patient education, with its profound impact on health care economics, is a multidimensional endeavor. Addressing these economic challenges, ethical dilemmas, and cultural considerations is not only essential for financial sustainability but also for maintaining ethical standards and promoting equitable health care. Navigating this complex terrain necessitates a comprehensive approach that recognizes the intricate relationship between patient education, economics, and the overall well-being of patients and health care systems.

FUTURE DIRECTIONS AND OPPORTUNITIES

Future research focused on the economics of health education should continue to emphasize the role of health care professional education and better utilization of current technology such as electronic health records (EHRs), telemedicine, and a universal system for health information exchange (HIE). The Health Information Technology for Economic and Clinical Health Act was signed into law in 2009 in support of health care reform to improve the utilization of EHRs and support the development of HIE.[20] Over a decade later, both have failed to meet their potential goals. Emerging trends such as smart technology and the advent of artificial intelligence (AI) should be explored as an adjunct for the improvement of health education and economics. The ultimate goal is to empower patients to be autonomous and accountable for their own health education with oversight from a health care professional. Financial benefits associated with health education also requires changing how health education is delivered to decrease the associated costs of printed material, translation services, and multimedia advertisements. Before the health care industry moves toward what will be in the future of medicine, it is imperative to continue to improve upon the foundation and fundamental building blocks of medicine that already exist.

Training Health Care Professionals

Of course, how we train the trainer will determine the effectiveness and quality of health education delivery, health economics, and ultimately patient outcomes.[4] In order to effectively bill for health education, training for health care professionals should be 3 fold. First, health care providers must be taught how to deliver culturally-competent education to patients at the appropriate level of education.[4] Second, patient education must be supported with documentation to facilitate appropriate billing. Lastly, to obtain the financial benefits for educational services, the level of coding must coincide with the provider's verbal education, which includes the amount of time spent educating the patient.

Electronic Health Records

To err is human, and electronic medical records (EHRs) have played a significant role in minimizing and eliminating human error to increase the quality of health care delivered.[20] For example, medication errors have decreased with proper use of an EHR with prepopulated medication names, doses, route, and directions that include electronic signatures that can be conveniently transmitted electronically directly to the patent's pharmacy of choice. EHRs also provide a certain level of autonomy for patients by allowing access to their personal health information. This allows increased accessibility to the health care provider between scheduled visits as well as the means to request appointments, medications, and patient education in real time. The caveat to the EHR is the patient must have some level of health literacy, most often speak, read, and write in English, and have access to a personal computer or smart phone. With the continued use of the EHRs, however, we have created another platform in which the provider can provide health education but may not be receiving the financial benefits of doing so. This missed opportunity can be associated with a lack of provider documentation, coding, or billing for patient education that may not be captured outside of the usual in-person office visits.

Health Information Exchange

The search for a universal HIE appears to be a tireless and never-ending journey for the health care industry.[21] Long awaited is an electronic platform that links each organization's individualized medical software system to integrate patient information and patient care between health professionals while enforcing the level of protection and privacy at or above its current level.[21,22] The evolution of an HIE is warranted but has yet to come to fruition. The current demand for such a system has yet to be proved greater than the challenges associated with its inception. More importantly, the economic benefits may have yet to be calculated but can easily be imagined, for example, less need for duplicate laboratories, imaging, and improved efficiency through HIE to support care coordination.[14]

Emerging Trends

Smart technologies

The use of smart technology is an emerging trend that supports health education, health literacy, patient accountability and proves to be economically beneficial. Wearable devices such as personal smart watches or glucose monitoring systems are 2 examples of such smart technologies that give real-time feedback at a fraction of the cost when compared to traditional practices.[23] Health care providers can also utilize remote monitoring as a source of immediate intervention, which prevents delay in care, improves overall health outcomes, and decreases the financial burden of inefficiencies for both the patient and the health care institution.[23] Software applications continue to serve as the monitoring system of smart technologies; however, standardization should be prioritized to ensure they meet the same level of protection and privacy as similar medical software that proceeded their existence.

The integration of telemedicine supports the use of smart technology and can be integrated into health education for both the provider and patient. Telemedicine can also solve access to health care issues, decreasing patient wait time while increasing the delivery of care without simultaneously increasing the associated overhead cost associated with staffing and the use of medical supplies require for in-person visits such as gloves and gowns. Increased utilization of telemedicine can make current resources go further and benefit health systems economically. Despite advances in technology, there continues to be an underutilization and lack of standardization of telemedicine, which minimizes the infinite possibilities of its economical benefits. One must take note that although technology is available and accessible, all are not technology savvy. There is a learning curve that both patient and provider must obtain to benefit what technology offers in the delivery of efficient and effective care. The macrocosm of long-term benefits in health education and health economics can only be measured once an integrated HIE truly exists between all health care systems.

Artificial intelligence

AI utilizes technology to complete task that typically require human intelligence, discernment, and decision-making through algorithms predefined rules and pattern recognition.[14] The role of AI in multiple disciplines continues to be on the rise.[24] The integration of AI appears to be inevitable in health care, but there continue to be gaps in the literature in how to maximize its utilization and where it will create the greatest impact.[25] Utilized in conjunction with telemedicine, AI can transform documentation, increasing efficiency in provider or nurse charting, billing, and developing and deploying patient education across languages and in forms that patients can access long after they leave the provider's office. Once in place, one must also question how AI will be monitored is such a diverse, complex, and constantly changing health care system. Despite these unknowns, the advent of AI can exponentially improve health economics and bring health education to a level beyond what is humanly possible.

Recommendations

Outside of the health care realm, legislators, stakeholders, and community leaders play an integral role in making short-term ideas manifest into long-term commitments in eliminating SDoHs through economic policy. Eliminating SDoHs addresses the challenges of health literacy.[5,8] Legislation that supports health education programs to minimize health literacy become long-term goals supported by economic policy. According to Sayer, economic policy can eliminate SDoHs by developing programs that recognize health inequalities and address them through the equitable dissemination of economic resources.[26] This concept is supported by Shipton, who believes health inequalities are deeply interwoven in our economic structure; therefore, to address the latter, one must eliminate the former.[27]

Future research should take a wholistic approach toward the short-term and long-term benefits associated with the economics of health education. Efforts must be made to explore the complexity of health from training health professionals that include crucial communications, cultural, social, and financial constructs that impede economic growth. Lastly, there is a political component that intertwines health and finances that exist and must be unveiled through legislation and economic policy.

SUMMARY

Despite the need for further research in health economics, which begins in the medical training phase, providers will ultimately develop their own style in the delivery of health education. Simultaneously, programs must be created to monitor, access, and ensure health education is appropriately reimbursed and supported through economic policy. There has been a paradigm shift in health education from one that is solely provider-led to one that involves patient-centered care and shared decision-making to improve health outcomes that can result in financial benefits. Although the economics of health education is initiated at the practice and organizational level, long-term benefits must be conducted globally with standardization, monitoring, and appropriate oversight.

Providers and patients require some level of health and financial literacy to acquire the economic benefits associated with health education. Improving health literacy starts with addressing language, communication, cultural, social, and economic barriers to support effective health education.[5,6,9] Financial literacy entails understanding how medical services for a patient are financially covered and how the provider will be reimbursed for such services.[14] Providers should participate in continuing medical education that supports accurate coding and effective billing to reap the financial benefits in a climate that is constantly changing to meet the demands of the health care industry. Health education promotes wellness, minimizes morbidity and mortality, and may be the missing link in minimizing hospitalizations and hospital readmissions that can result in billions of dollars annually.[6,9]

Given the complex interplay between patient education and economic outcomes, more rigorous studies on cost–benefit analysis are warranted to better quantify these relationships and inform policy and practice.

CLINICS CARE POINTS

- Personalized, theory-driven patient education is needed in order to enhance health outcomes and support financial sustainability.
- SDoHs and health literacy can influence the economic benefits of health promotion and disease prevention.

- Effective patient education begins with evidence-based practices during the medical training phase for health care professionals.
- Patients and health care professionals must improve their health and financial literacy to optimize the economic benefits of health education.

CASE STUDY
Case Study 13.1 Fee Schedule

Scenario: A 46 year old woman with no known past medical history, with new diagnosis of type 2 diabetes mellitus found with a blood glucose of 300 mg/dL and a hemoglobin A1c of 10.3%. Despite the US$100 office charge, the Medicare approved fee schedule only allows a maximum of US$75 reimbursement for the services provided. Medicare will pay 80% (US$60) of the fee schedule and the patient is responsible for paying 20% (US$15). Any amount charged to the patient exceeding the Medicare fee schedule would need to be written off by the practice (US$100 – US$75 = US$25).

Services Provided	Office Charge	Medicare Fee Schedule
Diabetes education (15 min)	US$100	US$75
Medicare payment	Patient payment	Practice write-off
US$60 (80%)	US$15 (20%)	US$25

Note: Scenario assumes the provider participates in Medicare and the patient has met the financial responsibility of their deductible.

Diabetes education may consist of patient management to begin insulin pump therapy (also called continuous subcutaneous insulin infusion or CSII) as it relates to insulin, such as carb ratios, basal rates, sick day management, or insulin sensitivity for correction factor. Medical nutrition therapy specifically focuses on dietary intervention to ensure eating habits are appropriate for persons with diabetes. For Medicare, diabetes self-management training and medical nutrition therapy are completely separate benefits.

CPT Code[3]	Description	Providers Who Can Perform the Service	CY 2023 Total RVUs (Nonfacility)[5]	CY 2023 Medicare National Rate[5]	Notes
Diabetes Education by Physician or Equivalent Practitioner					
99202	Office or other outpatient visit for the evaluation and management of a new patient, which requires a medically appropriate history and/or examination and straightforward medical decision making. When using time for code selection, 15–29 min of total time is spent on the date of the encounter.	Physician (MD, DO) Physician Assistant (PA) Nurse Practitioner (NP) Clinical Nurse Specialist (CNS)	2.15	$73	Physicians and equivalents report E/M codes for education services that they personally perform.
99203	Office or other outpatient visit for the evaluation and management of a new patient, which requires a medically appropriate history and/or examination and low level of medical decision making. When using time for		3.33	$113	

(continued on next page)

(continued)

CPT Code[3]	Description	Providers Who Can Perform the Service	CY 2023 Total RVUs (Nonfacility)[5]	CY 2023 Medicare National Rate[5]	Notes
	code selection, 30–44 min of total time is spent on the date of the encounter.				
99204	Office or other outpatient visit for the evaluation and management of a new patient, which requires a medically appropriate history and/or examination and moderate level of medical decision making. When using time for code selection, 45–59 min of total time is spent on the date of the encounter.		4.94	$167	
99205	Office or other outpatient visit for the evaluation and management of a new patient, which requires a medically appropriate history and/or examination and high level of medical decision making. When using time for code selection, 60–74 min of total time is spent on the date of the encounter		6.52	$221	
99211	Office or other outpatient visit for the evaluation and management of an established patient, that may not require the presence of a physician or other qualified health care professional. Usually, the presenting problem(s) are minimal.		0.69	$23	
99212	Office or other outpatient visit for the evaluation and management of an established patient, which requires a medically appropriate history and/or examination and straightforward medical decision making. When using time for code selection, 10–19 min of total time is spent on the date of the encounter		1.68	$57	
99213	Office or other outpatient visit for the evaluation and management of an established patient, which requires a medically appropriate history and/or examination and low level of medical decision making. When using time for code selection, 20–29 min of total time is spent on the date of the encounter		2.68	$91	
99214	Office or other outpatient visit for the evaluation and management of an established patient, which requires a medically appropriate history and/or examination and moderate level of medical decision making. When using time for code selection, 30–39 min of total time is spent on the date of the encounter		3.79	$128	
99215	Office or other outpatient visit for the evaluation and management of an established patient, which requires a medically appropriate history and/or examination and high level of medical decision making. When using time for code selection, 40–54 min of total time is spent on the date of the encounter.		5.31	$180	

DISCLOSURE

The authors have nothing to disclose. T. Harris, DHA, MS, PA-C has no conflict of interest to declare. No financial support was provided in the preparation of this article. L. Okolie, DMSc, MBA, MHS, PA-C has no conflict of interest to declare. No financial support was provided in the preparation of this article.

REFERENCES

1. Paterick TE, Patel N, Tajik AJ, et al. Improving health outcomes through patient education and partnerships with patients. Bayl Univ Med Cent 2017;30(1):112–3.
2. Callender LDR, Johnson AD, Pignataro RP. Patient-centered education in wound management: improving outcomes and adherence. Adv Skin Wound Care 2021; 34(8):1.
3. CDC. Health and economic costs of chronic diseases. Centers for Disease Control and Prevention. 2023. Available at: https://www.cdc.gov/chronicdisease/about/costs/index.htm. [Accessed 20 April 2024].
4. Hivert MF, McNeil A, Lavie CJ, et al. Training health professionals to deliver healthy living medicine. Prog Cardiovasc Dis 2017;59(5):471–8.
5. Cabellos-García AC, Castro-Sánchez E, Martínez-Sabater A, et al. Relationship between determinants of health, equity, and dimensions of health literacy in patients with cardiovascular disease. Int J Environ Res Publ Health 2020;17(6): 2082.
6. Nutbeam D. From health education to digital health literacy - building on the past to shape the future. Glob Health Promot 2021;28(4):51–5.
7. Ranasinghe PD, Pokhrel S, Anokye NK. Economics of physical activity in low-income and middle- income countries: a systematic review. BMJ Open 2021; 11(1):e037784.
8. Baek Y, Ademi Z, Fisher J, et al. Equity in economic evaluations of early childhood development interventions in low-and middle-income countries: scoping review. Matern Child Health J 2023;27(6):1009–29.
9. Gentizon J, Bovet E, Rapp E, et al. Medication literacy in hospitalized older adults: concept development. Health Lit Res Pract 2022;6(2):e70–83.
10. Luther B, Wilson RD, Kranz C, et al. Discharge processes: what evidence tells us is most effective. Orthop Nurs 2019;38(5):328–33.
11. Lakerveld J, Palmeira AL, van Duinkerken E, et al. Motivation: key to a healthy lifestyle in people with diabetes? Current and emerging knowledge and applications. Diabet Med 2020;37(3):464–72.
12. Pardo G, Pineda ED, Ng CD, et al. The association between persistence and adherence to disease-modifying therapies and healthcare resource utilization and costs in patients with multiple sclerosis. J Health Econ Outcomes Res 2022;9(1):111–6.
13.. Feldman MD, Christensen JF. Behavioral medicine: a guide for clinical practice. 4th edition. New York, NY: McGraw Hill Education; 2014.
14. Devlin AM, McCormack G. Physician responses to medicare reimbursement rates. J Health Econ 2023;92:102816.
15. Geruso M, Richards MR. Trading spaces: Medicare's regulatory spillovers on treatment setting for non-medicare patients. J Health Econ 2022;84:102624.
16. Conway A, Satin D. The role of pay-for-performance in reducing healthcare disparities: a narrative literature review. Prev Med 2022;164:107274.
17. Mantwill S, Monestel-Umaña S, Schulz PJ. The relationship between health literacy and health disparities: a systematic review. PLoS One 2015;10(12):e0145455.

18. Katz P, Dall'Era M, Trupin L, et al. Impact of limited health literacy on patient-reported outcomes in systemic lupus erythematosus. Arthritis Care Res 2021; 73(1):110–9.
19. Smith ML, Zhong L, Lee S, et al. Effectiveness and economic impact of a diabetes education program among adults with type 2 diabetes in South Texas. BMC Publ Health 2021;21:1646.
20. Mills S. Electronic health records and use of clinical decision support. Crit Care Nurs Clin North Am 2019;31(2):125–31.
21. Holmgren AJ, Adler-Milstein J. Health Information Exchange in US Hospitals: the current landscape and a path to improved information sharing. J Hosp Med 2017; 12(3):193–8.
22. Moore W, Frye S. Review of HIPAA, Part 1: history, protected health information, and privacy and security rules. J Nucl Med Technol 2019;47(4):269–72.
23. Ullah M, Hamayun S, Wahab A, et al. Smart technologies used as smart tools in the management of cardiovascular disease and their future perspective [published online ahead of print, 2023 Jul 10]. Curr Probl Cardiol 2023;48(11):101922.
24. Howard J. Artificial intelligence: implications for the future of work. Am J Ind Med 2019;62(11):917–26.
25. Chen M, Decary M. Artificial intelligence in healthcare: an essential guide for health leaders. Healthc Manage Forum 2020;33(1):10–8.
26. Sayer A, McCartney G. Economic relationships and health inequalities: improving public health recommendations. Publ Health 2021;199:103–6.
27. Shipton D, Sarica S, Craig N, et al. Knowing the goal: an inclusive economy that can address the public health challenges of our time. J Epidemiol Community Health 2021;75(11):1129–32.

Preparing Physician Assistant/Associate Students for Patient Education

Justina Bennett, MPAS, PA-C

KEYWORDS

- Physician Assistant (PA) students • Patient education • Affective learning domain
- Emotional intelligence • Shared decision-making • Provider–patient relationship

KEY POINTS

- Affective learning domain concepts such as interpersonal and communication skills are crucial to provider–patient relationships.
- Emotional intelligence competencies include active listening, interpreting others' emotions via verbal and nonverbal cues, and practicing empathy.
- Didactive teaching, role play with simulated patients, and direct faculty feedback displaying emotional intelligence to the physician assistant/associate (PA) student significantly improves student confidence in providing patient education.
- Communication, teamwork, and leadership skills are fostered by emotional intelligence and social competence in PA students leading to organizational awareness allowing multiple professions to seek common goals such as providing effective patient education.

INTRODUCTION

Patient education is defined as "the process by which the patient comes to comprehend his or her physical condition and self-care by the use of various medians and experiences."[1] Patient education is one of the great opportunities in medicine to actively participate in a conversation that has the potential to change the course of a patient's life. With well-taught patient education, the patients can leave their health care encounter empowered and inspired to take the correct steps to move in the direction of healthier living. The shared act of patient education between the health care provider (HCP) and the patient is a combination of both the art and the science of medicine[2] as well as effective communication and understanding between the 2 parties.[3]

In this article, the authors highlight how to prepare physician assistant/associate (PA) students to provide patient education. The authors focus on the essential skills required for effective patient education, teaching strategies and methods for

Department of PA Medicine, Frostburg State University, 24 N. Walnut Street, Hagerstown, MD 21740, USA
E-mail addresses: jabennett@frostburg.edu; Justina.Olsen@hotmail.com

Physician Assist Clin 9 (2024) 633–641
https://doi.org/10.1016/j.cpha.2024.05.012
2405-7991/24/© 2024 Elsevier Inc. All rights are reserved, including those for text and data mining, AI training, and similar technologies.

physicianassistant.theclinics.com

educating PA students on the delivery of patient education as well as the importance of interprofessional collaboration and team-based approaches to providing patient education. Patient education is part of the standard of care for all HCPs who interact with patients, including PA students.[2]

BACKGROUND AND CONTEXT

The patient education health promotion model combines many concepts of the self-efficacy model and acknowledges that patient behavior is affected by many factors and influences all of which are unique to the individual and thus must be understood by the health care professional.[1] This model mirrors the shift in medicine from a paternalistic to a patient-centered approach to care. Patient education, much like all aspects of medicine, is not a "one-size-fits-all" but rather must be tailored to the individual to be the most effective and meaningful.[2] Therefore, effective interpersonal and communication skills are a crucial component of this interaction between the HCP and the patient and thus must be present in PA education.[3–5] Interpersonal and communication skills fall under the affective learning domain while cognitive and psychomotor learning domains are the most readily addressed in PA education. Medical knowledge easily falls under the cognitive domain and physical examination and procedural skills are within the psychomotor domain. The affective domain is often neglected in health professions education but is crucial for patient interactions and relationships, perhaps most notably defined in providing meaningful patient education.[6]

Historically, communication was not formally "taught" but addressed during the clinical years of medical education via faculty feedback on actual patient interactions.[3] These skills were often acquired naturally during clinical experiences, but it was thought that these skills should be "strengthened and organized for increased efficiency and effectiveness" early on in health professions education.[5] However, without a standardized approach, there were significant gaps in a health profession students' ability to provide effective patient education which we know is crucial to best patient outcomes. The Advisory Committee on Training in Primary Care Medicine now recommends that health professions education programs should provide training specific to giving patient education via shared-medical decision-making that leads to improved patient outcomes.[7] The Association of American Medical Colleges recommends medical students learn communication techniques and then demonstrate how to use these techniques in patient interactions, including motivational interviewing.[4] This is encompassed in the professional competencies for PAs that include effective and appropriate application of medical knowledge, interpersonal and communication skills, patient care, professionalism, practice-based learning and improvement, and system-based practice.[8]

THEORETIC FOUNDATIONS

Bloom and colleagues developed the 3 learning categories that include cognitive, affective, and psychomotor domains.[6] The affective domain was further defined to include 5 core components (**Box 1**).[6] The affective domain represents skills that foster appropriate emotional responses [to patients] and thus require emotional intelligence. Emotional intelligence encompasses an intrapersonal and interpersonal intelligence that gives humans the ability to understand themselves and others.[9] It includes self-awareness, self-management, social awareness, and relationship management.[5] It is crucial in the development of skills such as time management, decision-making, accountability, empathy, presentation skills, stress tolerance, trust, and communication,[5] all essential in PA students and HCPs providing patient interactions and

> **Box 1**
> **Components of the affective learning domain[6]**
>
> Receiving—respectful listening, active listening
>
> Responding—engaging in interaction with others
>
> Valuing—ability to judge the worth/value of something
>
> Organizing—ability to compare, classify, and prioritize values and reconcile conflicting values
>
> Characterizing—establishment of a value system to allow personalization and independence

education. These components need to be implemented and evaluated early in PA students' education for improved patient-education interactions.[6]

In addition to the affective learning domain, it is important to note that both PA students and patients are adult learners. These learners are internally motivated, they want to know why they need to know something before starting the learning process, they are self-directed and take responsibility for their decisions, and they possess life experience that can enrich their learning but also requires individualization of learning strategies for this reason.[1] While PA students and patients are self-directed and autonomous, it is still crucial that teaching regarding providing patient education includes structure, instruction, and guidance as a partnership is cultivated with the patient.[1] The following will outline the current theory and components of teaching PA students to implement patient education to lead to best outcomes.

BEST PRACTICES AND STRATEGIES

Current research suggests that teaching and fostering interpersonal skills and emotional intelligence are a large part of teaching PA students how to not only effectively relay patient education but also how to improve the provider–patient encounter.[5,9] Educators in non-health care domains have stated that emotional intelligence is an essential competency for effective teaching. The same should hold true as we train PA students, future HCPs, to be "teachers of health" to patients.[9] Studies show that HCPs with emotional intelligence display empathy, respect, and genuineness.[9] They are more aware of patient's emotions that leads to improved patient outcomes by listening to patient's words, paying attention to nonverbal behavior, and empathizing with the patients by understanding their concerns and emotions.[9] Goleman noted that "the main competency of a person with emotional intelligence was a service orientation."[9] Emotional intelligence competencies are summarized in **Box 2**. These skills are necessary for the delivery of patient education and for the provider–patient relationship.

Active listening includes establishing eye contact and being fully present with the patient throughout an encounter.[3,9] Studies have shown that physicians interrupt

> **Box 2**
> **Emotional intelligence competencies[9]**
>
> Active listening
>
> Ability to read other individual's emotions including nonverbal behavior
>
> Empathizes by understanding concerns and emotions

patients in their opening statements in over half of visits just 18 to 23 seconds into the conversation.[3] Focusing on patient-centered interviewing skills by starting the encounter off with an open-ended question demonstrates a shift of power to allow the patient to feel that they are actively participating and are empowered in their health care. After the patient-centered interview process is complete, then the HCP can move into the provider-centered portion of the interview, but care needs to be taken to ensure that during direct questioning, eye contact is maintained allowing the patient to continue to be the focus of the encounter.[3] Reading and interpreting the patient's body language and controlling one's own body language is a crucial part of the encounter and plays a large role in the outcome.[3] Showing empathy, which is now included as an educational objective for medical training, is key and accomplished by active listening and demonstrating to patients that their concerns were heard.[3] A large part of evaluating education that focuses on the affective domain, and emotional intelligence competencies, is student reflection and revision.[6] Thus, opportunities should be given in the didactic and clinical year for the PA student to receive feedback specific to these emotional intelligence competencies. Demonstration of emotional intelligence by faculty is perhaps one of the most powerful teachers of affective skills. Studies have shown that active participation by the educator including regular, constructive feedback, and positive relational interactions with the PA student is crucial to the development and refinement of these skills.[6]

A stepwise approach should be part of the instruction for PA students as they approach patient interactions and education. The steps of the provider–patient interaction process are listed in **Box 3**. While step 1 of this list also involves the cognitive domain, steps 1 to 4 encompass the affective learning domain and the emotional intelligence competencies detailed earlier.

To develop effective teaching strategies and methods for educating PA students on the delivery of patient education, we need to understand what current evidenced-based research states is essential to providing effective patient education. The most effective patient education is individualized and patient-centered which follows the theory of the health promotion model.[1,2] Just as treatment plans are not a "one-size-fits-all" neither is patient education. Shared decision-making is a key component in the patient education process linked to high-quality patient education.[10] Shared decision-making includes the sharing of relevant information, the patient and the provider expressing treatment preferences, deliberating the options and agreement between the patient and the provider on the treatment to implement (**Box 4**).[10] Steps 1 and 2 of this process focus on the emotional intelligence competencies detailed previously. Steps 3 through 5 focus on tailoring patient education to the individual. This considers the patients' beliefs about themselves and the surrounding world, their

---

Box 3
Steps of provider–patient interaction[9]

Step 1: Provider explains disease, results, and plan

Step 2: Provider helps patient express emotions, beliefs, and expectations with empathy

Step 3: Providers show respect for values and preferences of the patient giving them the option to choose and make decisions for themselves after receiving education from the provider

Step 4: Effective communication makes the patient feel their decision is important

Step 5: Patient feels satisfied with the provider interaction

> **Box 4**
> **Strategies to teach physician assistant/associate students on how to improve provider–patient communication[3,10]**
>
> Step 1: Build a relationship ("active partnership")
>
> Step 2: Focus on listening
>
> Step 3: Collaborate on the treatment plan ("shared decision-making")
>
> Step 4: Manage time
>
> Step 5: Implement effective follow-up interventions

support network, their environment including social determinants of health—which may include factors such as education level, income, employment, housing, transportation, and access to healthy necessities (food, water, air), their level of emotional distress, and their mastery of needed skills.[1]

The 4 main components of patient education include assessment, planning, implementation, and evaluation.[2]

Assessment

How do we teach PA students to perform assessment? A large component of assessment is the emotional intelligence competency of active listening. PA students need to know the patients' perspective and knowledge of their situation. It is important to not only assess those regulatory requirements routinely captured on intake such as motivation to learn, religious/cultural beliefs, emotional barriers, cognitive/physical limitations, and communication barriers but also to ask "what are you most worried about?"[2] This question allows the HCP to see where the patients stand in their knowledge and perspective of the health care situation at hand and work to build the relationship between the provider and patient which in turn aids in the effectiveness of future education provided.[2] This harkens back to the health promotion model, the self-efficacy model, and more recently the explanatory model of patient education.[1,11] The explanatory model asserts that the patients' beliefs and social context greatly influence their ability to understand, manage, and prioritize their health.[11] Health literacy is key during the assessment process to ensure that communication is understood and successful. Health literacy is defined as "the degree to which individuals have the capacity to obtain, process, and understand basic health information and services needed to make appropriate health decisions."[2] Low health literacy is associated with age greater than 60 years, low income, low educational achievement, race (Black, Hispanic, American Indian/Native, and multiracial), those who did not speak English before formal education, those who rate their health as poor, use of public insurance or no insurance, and those who seek out health information less often.[2] Cutilli states there is no "gold standard" health literacy screening tool leading most often to overestimation of health literacy by HCPs.[2] Therefore, the concept of the Health Literacy Universal Precautions recommends to educate patients as if they have low health literacy.[2] Motivational interviewing also helps achieve these assessment goals when teaching PA students about the first step in patient education. It encompasses eliciting what motivates a patient to make health behavioral changes and incorporates empathy, nonjudgmental open-ended questions, and reflective listening to explore the patient's point of view, sharing many of the same concepts with emotional intelligence.

Planning and Implementation

The planning and implementation portions of patient education are accomplished together. Planning is directed by the assessment portion of the process.[2] When planning, it is important to consider format, language, and level of health literacy. Techniques of providing education may change depending on the topic, for example, if learning about medications, then reading or listening may be preferable, but if needing instruction on wound care or dressing changes, then demonstration may be the better choice.[2] Teaching methods are typically verbal or written. Verbal education should use language that is familiar to the patient avoiding medical terminology, teach the most important information first, make information as simple as possible without losing meaning, chunk information into short sections, use short words and sentences, and leave pauses in the conversation for patient reflection.[2] Written education uses similar strategies as verbal education but categorizes strategies as understandable and actionable.[2] Research indicates that implementation with multiple techniques of delivery is most effective and tailoring methods of implementation to individual needs and desires improves efficacy.[2] In addition to the format of patient education, other considerations include utilizing the patient's preferred language and simple repetitive instructions.[2] PA students should be given the opportunity, particularly in the clinical year, to observe and practice these various implementation modalities. This will allow them to further broaden their ability to convey patient education in ways that are understandable to patients.

Evaluation

Evaluation is the final component of the patient education process but is often given little attention. It is not simply asking "do you understand" but rather implementing various techniques such as knowledge tests, patient demonstration, and teach-back method to ensure the patient's understanding and allowing the opportunity to reteach patient education if necessary.[2]

A practical way to implement teaching these skills was demonstrated by the Mayo Medical School. They implemented a course in their program titled Health Behavior Change Counseling that occurred during the didactic portion of their curriculum. The main outcomes of the course were to have students enhance their provider–patient communication skills and to learn and practice motivational interviewing.[4] The students participated in 5 sessions that encompassed lectures and video examples on the basic concepts of motivational interviewing, active learning utilizing case vignettes and role play, and direct faculty feedback.[4] The curriculum started with detailing the basic concepts of motivational interviewing while comparing them to other counseling styles such as confrontational and nondirective interviewing.[4] There was a focus on differentiating between open-ended and closed-ended questions and reflective listening was discussed and practiced.[4] Students who completed the course affirmed that using didactive teaching, role play with simulated patients, and direct faculty feedback significantly improved their confidence in providing counseling to patients.[4]

Interprofessional collaboration and team-based approaches have positive effects on the delivery of patient education. Vijn and colleagues reviewed multiple studies in which medical students at various stages of their education (including undergraduate medical education, years 1–4) were utilized to provide education to patients. He found benefits to both medical students and patients when students delivered education. Medical students contributed effectiveness, accessibility, and equitable health care to patients.[12] Benefits to the students included enhancement of their communication skills, relations with patients, and patient education skills involving self-efficacy and behavior.[12] By fostering emotional intelligence and social competence in PA students, communication, teamwork, and leadership skills are developed which lead to organizational awareness.[9] Organizational awareness allows a range of people across professions to become motivated to seek the common objectives of providing quality and effective patient education and positively contribute to teamwork in the health care field.[9]

CHALLENGES AND CONSIDERATIONS

For those working in PA education, it is well known that time, or lack thereof, is the biggest constraint in the didactic curriculum. The didactic year is spent building upon clinical anatomy and physiology, teaching core clinical medicine concepts, physical examination, procedures, and the basis of clinical pharmacology. Simulation of all possible scenarios for patient education is near impossible as patient needs, and provider qualities are varied when it comes to all the nuances that may be encountered. Early assessment and development of emotional intelligence competencies in the didactic year of PA education are warranted to develop a set of underlying skills necessary to meet all the various nuances that each individual patient encounter may present. While development of the affective domain is time-consuming and requires specific types of teaching methods detailed previously, the long-term benefits to the students as well as future patients are great.[6] Additionally, the complexity of the learning outcomes associated with this topic can be challenging to evaluate and quantify but can be achieved through student reflection, direct instructor feedback shared with demonstration of emotional intelligence, and opportunity for revision by the student.[6]

In addition to these academic barriers in the didactic year of PA education, the clinical world is fraught with constraints. The widespread availability of medical information at patient's fingertips has altered the HCP role from "keeper of the medical information" to "interpreter and integrator of health care information for patients requiring affective skills and emotional intelligence."[3,9] The relationship between HCP and patient has been hindered in multiple ways as medicine has become more business-like with limited time during office visits and a larger focus on integrating technology which can be a barrier for some HCPs taking away from the patient interaction itself as well as precepting students.[3,9]

Vijn and colleagues showed that the literature confirms benefits of having undergraduate students interested in a health profession participate actively with patients in a clinical experience in the workplace. It is useful not only to the student but the patients as well with data showing enhancement of patient disease knowledge, health attitude, health behavior, medication adherence, and disease management.[12] The same should hold true for PA students in their didactic year of education and continuing into their clinical year. Dedicated time for a clinical experience and during clinical experiences with a focus on practicing emotional intelligence competencies, specifically as they relate to providing patient education, through an internship, service-learning education requirement, or a student-run clinic would be valuable.[12]

Bhattad and colleagues found barriers to patient education that included an insufficient number of HCPs trained to provide patient education, overall inexperience of HCPs with providing patient education, high turnover of HCPs, and limited time for HCPs to give patient education.[7] PA educators are poised to meet these first 2 challenges by intentionally making space in the didactic and clinical years to implement opportunities to learn the skills required, the components of patient education process, and practice implementation of that process. Providing space to discuss other barriers to patient education including health literacy,[2] language and cultural issues, and support system[10] throughout the didactic and clinical years of PA education could be directly tied to the improvement of patient education delivery and patient care as well.

FUTURE DIRECTIONS AND OPPORTUNITIES

It is no surprise that patient outcomes improve with a healthy provider–patient relationship, ideally first found in a primary care setting. This is evidenced in the recent American health care story and primary care crisis resulting in the overall declining health of the population.[13] It also rings true where patient education is concerned. Using emotional intelligence competencies that have been taught and refined during medical education, we need to train students to build these relationships with patients because the goal of patient education is to aid the patients in changing their behavior and that is best done in the context of a longitudinal relationship.[9] Our colleagues in the marketing world have captured this as is evidenced in the book *Selling the Invisible*.[2] The author notes that in the service industry, the key to success is building relationships.[2] Certain marketing techniques such as making patient education a simple basic message, inserting an "unexpected aspect" to make the content memorable and relevant to the patient, conveying concrete and clear ideas, giving credible information, involving emotion in the encounter, and giving patient education as a narrative or a story have all been proposed to help patient education "stick" or translate into changed behavior and healthier living.[2] Lastly, and perhaps best suited to the provider–patient relationship model, multiple sources suggest that information is best received and remembered when it is presented in a way that fits into the patient's worldview.[2] Future opportunities for PA students and providers to give patient education are present and needed in all specialties of medicine. They have the greatest impact when provided in a primary care setting due to the unique longstanding nature of the relationship and the maximal influence that it can have on patient's choices.[13]

SUMMARY

The interaction between the patients and provider has long been held as sacred. The relationship is complex and rich, and as we train PA students, it is important to educate them not only on the cognitive and psychomotor skills necessary to provide quality care but also the affective skills needed to nurture the partnership and provide patients with education to promote healthier living. Reframing the interaction into one of services to the patients sets the stage for building upon emotional intelligence. Emotional intelligence is key to recognize that we are each, provider and patient, bringing our experiences, values, and emotions to the table. We will only be successful at improving health at the individual and population level when we can engage in a meaningful genuine relationship dedicated to mutual respect and caring.

CLINICS CARE POINTS

- Competencies of emotional intelligence are key in giving effective patient education and these include active listening, the ability to read other individual's emotions including their nonverbal behavior and empathizing by understanding concerns and emotions.
- Effective comunication and shared decision making are key for patient-provider satisfaction.

- Major barriers to teaching physician assistant students how to give effective patient education include time constraints during didactic education, time constraints during clinical encounters, lack of experience and health literacy of patients.

DISCLOSURE

The author has no conflicts of interest.

REFERENCES

1. Syx RL. The practice of patient education. Orthop Nurs 2008;27(1):50–6. PMID: 18300691.
2. Cutilli CC. Excellence in patient education: evidence-based education that "sticks" and improves patient outcomes. Nurs Clin North Am 2020;55(2):267–82.
3. Teutsch C. Patient - doctor communication. Med Clin North Am 2003;87:1115–45.
4. Poirier MK, Clark MM, Cerhan JH, et al. Teaching motivational interviewing to first-year medical students to improve counseling skills in health behavior change. Mayo Clin Proc 2004;79:327–31.
5. Khademi E, Abdi M, Saeidi M, et al. Emotional intelligence and quality of nursing care: A need for continuous professional development. Iran J Nurs Midwifery Res 2021;26(4):361–7.
6. Wu WH, Kao HY, Wu SH, et al. Development and evaluation of affective domain using student's feedback in entrepreneurial Massive Open Online Courses. Front Psychol 2019;1109(10):1–9.
7. Bhattad PB, Pacifico L. Empowering patients: promoting patient education and health literacy. Cureus 2022;14(7):1–15.
8. Competencies for the Physician Assistant Profession. 2013. Available at: https://www.aapa.org/wp-content/uploads/2017/02/PA-Competencies-updated.pdf#:~:text=Professional%20competencies%20for%20physician%20assistants%20include%20the%20effective,professionalism%2C%20practice-based%20learning%20and%20improvement%2C%20and%20syste. [Accessed 27 April 2024].
9. Omid A, Haghani F, Adibi P. Emotional intelligence: an old issue and a new look in clinical teaching. Adv Biomed Res 2018;7(1):1–6.
10. Bukstein DA. Patient adherence and effective communication. Ann Allergy Asthma Immunol 2016;117(6):613–9.
11. Bokhour BG, Cohn ES, Cortés DE, et al. The role of patients' explanatory models and daily-lived experience in hypertension self-management. J Gen Intern Med 2012;27(12):1626–34.
12. Vijn TW, Fluit CRMG, Kremer JAM, et al. Involving medical students in providing patient education for real patients: a scoping review. J Gen Intern Med 2017;32(9):1031–43.
13. Marcadis AR, Marti JL, Ehdaie B, et al. Characterizing relative and disease-specific survival in early-stage cancers. JAMA Intern Med 2020;180(3):461–3.

Ethical Considerations and Future Directions in Patient Education

Jeanine Gargiulo, MPAS, PA-C[a],
James F. Cawley, MPH, PA-C Emeritus, DHL(Hon)[b,c],*

KEYWORDS

- Patient education • Biomedical ethics • Provider–patient relationship
- Personalized medicine

KEY POINTS

- New concepts regarding patient education are emerging, and now relationship building is the cornerstone of excellent patient care.
- The struggle over a patient's role in medical decision-making is often characterized as a conflict between autonomy and health, between the values of a patient and the values of a physician.
- Spiritualty has been recognized as a key factor in health care. It is a broad concept that may affect not only end-of-life care but every aspect of patient health care. There are many advantages to becoming familiar with a patient's spiritual desires and needs.
- Modern guidelines are often viewed as nonmalleable, but the beauty of personalized medicine in an educational sense includes patient preference, and sometimes, the best plan may stray from this worn path of processes.
- It is apparent that in order to incorporate patient preference, thorough patient education must be provided to ensure quality shared decision-making.

THE LAW AND ETHICS

The delivery of health care in the United States is governed by an assortment of rules, regulations, laws as well as ethical standards. There are differences between legal and ethical standards. Laws are intended to protect individuals when making decisions about their health care. In addition, laws specify the responsibilities and expected conduct of health care professionals. Legal standards are determined by governmental laws and are useful as they help people to understand what they are not

[a] Physician Assistant Program, Graduate School, University of Maryland, Baltimore, Baltimore, MD 21201, USA; [b] Physician Assistant Leadership and Learning Academy, University of Maryland Baltimore, Baltimore, MD, USA; [c] The George Washington University
* Corresponding author.
E-mail address: purljfc@aol.com

Physician Assist Clin 9 (2024) 643–653
https://doi.org/10.1016/j.cpha.2024.05.013   physicianassistant.theclinics.com
2405-7991/24/© 2024 Elsevier Inc. All rights reserved, including those for text and data mining, AI training, and similar technologies.

allowed to do. Ethical standards do not necessarily have a legal basis and are primarily based on human principles of right and wrong. With legal standards in place, authorities are allowed to enforce rules when people do something illegal, whereas ethical standards lack such regulation.

THE HEALING RELATIONSHIP AND PATIENT EDUCATION

Traditionally, the patient–health professional relationship has been structured around the utilitarian concept where a patient is seen as having a disease produced by either an external factor or a malfunctioning structure that is the source of pain, disability, or unhappiness. The recognition and treatment of a disease, if successful, will restore a patient's well-being. This clinical model underscores much of mainstream medical practice. Over the past few decades, patient autonomy has gradually replaced the paternalistic approach based on the premise that a physician knows what is best for a patient. Alternatively, the "relational model," a more recent incarnation, pertains to the quality of the process of the patient–physician interaction.[1] The struggle over a patient's role in medical decision-making is often characterized as a conflict between autonomy and health, between the values of a patient and the values of a physician. Seeking to curtail physician dominance, many have advocated an ideal of greater patient control.[2] This framework substitutes the health provider's role of being an expert providing technical expertise and knowledge to the patient who passively accepts with one where the relationship now becomes a partaking one for both players in the framework of which they exchange information. Based on the ethical principle of autonomy, a patient is transformed from a passive bystander into an active and integral participant in the healing process. Neither the paternalistic model of provider–patient relationship nor the informative model is considered to be totally satisfactory, as the paternalistic model excludes patient values from decision-making, while the informative model excludes physician values from decision-making. However, the deliberative model of patient–physician interaction represents an adequate alternative to the 2 unsatisfactory approaches by promoting shared decision-making between a physician and a patient. It has also been suggested that the deliberative model would be ideal for exercising patient autonomy in chronic care and that the ethical role of patient education would be to make the deliberative model applicable to chronic care.[3] In any joint relationship, and especially with a credence type of service, communication leading to mutual trust is a crucial element in the success of the interaction.

As practicing providers implement these changing models into their practice, broad socioeconomics should be considered. Specifically, in the relational model or deliberative model, verbal and written communication should be tailored to the patient to enable them to make an informed decision. Medical jargon must naturally be translated to layman's terms, but it also needs to be done with intention based on patient reading levels, educational background, primary language, and home and social support. An urban inner-city clinic may need to tailor their verbiage and patient education materials differently than a private practice who markets to patients in an affluent area of suburbia. While all of humanity requires medical attention, how clinicians provide the same care will likely appear different due to applying the aforementioned models.

Some challenges arise when the pendulum swings toward one of the extremes in the informative patient–providers relationship. If a patient is an extremist on the autonomy side, the challenging or "overinformed" patient can emerge. While patients who suffer from rare illnesses may truly be the expert compared to general practitioners, it is a rare scenario. More commonly, the overinformed patient can unintentionally undermine their own care. They may view the practitioner as solely the technical expert, and fully expect to have their medical values and decisions implemented, no matter the basis for their reasoning. What patients may fail to realize is medical providers have gained expertise based on preferences, their own research, and experiences. For example, a patient may come to a leading orthopedic joint replacement specialist demanding a specific type of joint replacement implant or technique. Consequently, veering off the standard protocols would likely increase risks and decrease the likelihood of a perfect outcome. Ethically, the surgeon should disclose their standard implants and techniques to the patient and explain that they are the expert in what they do every day. Patients may have a blind spot and plow through this knowledge with little regard for the facts in the educational component and physician values. These patients may also disregard other patient education or instructions and go rogue by manipulating their full control over their own care, completely ignoring any collaboration with the medical team. Classically, a specific socioeconomic status group stereotypically aligns with this overinformed patient. In all hyperinformed patients, their sources of knowledge acquisition to gain expertise must be examined and critiqued as well.

As more patients become actively involved in their care, there has been an evolution toward more thorough patient education. Patient and their advocates have pushed against a one-size-fits-all approach and instead desire a customized experience. An important current trend in health care that professionals must consider is medical decisions are becoming more standardized and codified. With this realization, it is important to be intentional with patient education and not base it or medical decision-making exclusively on formal guidelines. Decisions and directives need to be individualized, especially when they involve choices between possible outcomes that may be viewed differently by different patients.

It is interesting to note the differing perspectives of the involved parties in the physician–patient relationship. Patients traditionally stress the importance of the provider to offer effective interpersonal and communication skills.[4] In contrast, physicians stress the significance of the technical expertise and knowledge of health providers, emphasizing the role of competence and performance.[5] Physicians evaluate the relationship on the basis of their ability to solve problems through devotion, serviceability, reliability, and trustworthiness and disregard the "softer" interpersonal aspects such as caring, appreciation, and empathy that have been found to be important to their patients. This illustrates a mismatch in the important components of relationship building that can lead to a loss of trust, satisfaction, and repeat purchase.[3]

BASIC ETHICAL PRINCIPLES

The core ethical principles help guide health care professionals in making complex decisions and in maintaining a standard of care that prioritizes the well-being and rights of the patient. Adhering to these principles fosters a culture of trust, compassion, and professionalism within the health care system. Health care providers are often encouraged to undergo ongoing training and education in medical ethics to ensure that they can navigate difficult situations and provide the best possible care for their patients. The core principles of ethics are listed as follows:

Autonomy: Having respect for the right of the patient to make their own decisions regarding their health care and includes the right to refuse treatment.

Beneficence: It is a health professional's duty to act in the best interests of a patient.

Nonmaleficence: Avoiding actions that could harm a patient: the rule of "first, do no harm."

Justice: The assurance of fairness and equality in the utilization of health care resources and treatments regardless of race, gender, social status, or financial resources.

Additionally, there are several other ethical concepts that hold value in the provider–patient relationship.

Veracity: Honesty and truthfulness in communication with patients are critical in building trust in the provider–patient relationship.

Confidentiality: Respect for the privacy of patients in terms of their information regarding their condition, treatment, and potential outcomes is essential for a trusting provider–patient relationship.

Fidelity: Building and maintaining trust in the provider–patient relationship is based on honoring commitments and responsibilities.

Respect for dignity: A positive provider–patient relationship includes treating patients with respect, recognizing their worth as individuals.

PATIENT EDUCATION AND ETHICS

Ethical patient education practices, first of all, respect patient autonomy and dignity and seek to provide them with current and accurate information about their health conditions. This includes ensuring that patients understand their diagnoses, treatment options, and potential risks and benefits associated with each treatment option. It also permits patients to ask questions and receive honest answers in a confidential setting and to offer this information in a culturally competent manner. Ethical patient education practices help ensure that patients receive the best care possible. When patients are well-informed about their condition and treatment options, they are more likely to make decisions that are in their best interests.[6,7]

Patient education can be construed as being a widely encompassing term. To some, patient education is a specific set of communications often expressed in referrals and in writing. For others, patient education refers to the complexities of the provider–patient relationship and expressed through diagnoses, treatment directions and choices, and management options. It is also the case that effective and comprehensive patient education is facing new challenges in our fragmented and expensive health care system. Among the issues are the huge influx of patients of varying cultures and nationalities into the US health system, the lack of time available for providers to conduct an effective visit in limited scheduled managed care timeframes, the shortage of language-specific patient educational materials written at appropriate readability levels, and issues in fair reimbursement policies for time spent on patient education. Ethical dimensions applied to these types of issues in patient education include not only duty to the patient but also considerations of justice, respect for patient dignity, and veracity. Newer models of patient education have been proposed.[6] Historically, models of patient–provider interaction held that patient autonomy assumed that patients' medical knowledge was low. Unfortunately, this assumption has proven inadequate as it neither includes patients such as those who are highly educated nonmedical individuals who possesses little familiarity with health-related values but is highly autonomous nor includes patients from a non-Western background who may have well-established health care-related values but a low sense of personal independence. It is also evident that the assumption that all patients possess little medical knowledge is contradicted by those well-informed patients with a rare disease. An update to the models of Emanuel and Emanuel proposes a paradigm that models autonomy, health care-related values formation, and medical knowledge as varying from patient to patient.[8]

CODES OF ETHICAL CONDUCT

To provide ethical conduct guidelines, various health professions organizations have put forward codes of ethics. Probably, the best well known is the Code of Ethics of the American Medical Association (AMA), which is widely used and often-cited source of ethical advice.[9] Importantly, the AMA code notes in its preamble that ethical values and legal principles are closely related and that ethical responsibilities usually exceed legal duties. It observes further, "conduct that is legally permissible may be ethically unacceptable. Conversely, the fact that a physician who has been charged with allegedly illegal conduct has been acquitted or exonerated in criminal or civil proceedings does not necessarily mean that the physician acted ethically."[9] The American Academy of Physician Associates has adopted a code of ethics that is specific for physician associate, formerly named physician assistant (PA) providers. It's opening preamble states, "the PA profession has revised its code of ethics several times since the profession began. Although the fundamental principles underlying the ethical care of patients have not changed, the societal framework in which those principles are applied is constantly changing. Economic pressures, social pressures of church and state on the health care system, technological advances, and changing patient demographics continually transform the landscape in which PAs practice. This policy, as written, reflects a point in time and should be reviewed though that lens. It is a living document to be continually reviewed and updated to reflect the changing times, be they related to societal evolutions or the advancement of medical science."[10]

CULTURE AND COMMUNICATION

To provide true, well-rounded care, providers must think and practice beyond the commonly acknowledged values. Traditionally, these values are implemented with the end goal of healing or curing the patient. While there are areas of medicine focused on end-of-life care, it is often forgotten that common core values frequently lie between these two extreme patient scenarios. Perhaps spirituality should be discussed with the patient regularly and not just with a devastating diagnosis like cancer or chronic neurological disorder. True values that drive patient decision-making often lie in their spiritual beliefs. When a provider recognizes a patient's spiritual needs, they are seen as more compassionate and caring individuals. Various definitions of spirituality exist and application into the medical profession likely works best as incorporating a spiritual history. PA education programs have started to incorporate this spiritual history into the curriculum foundations of learning so the current student population who will comprise our future workforce of physician associates is well prepared to integrate this into clinical practice. The Association of American Medical Collages has a formal recommendation for implementing a curriculum on spirituality. The FICA method, outlined below in **Table 1**, is offered as a concise structure to utilize while gathering a patient's spiritual history.[11]

Spirituality has been studied with three areas of patient effect: mortality, coping, and recovery. The extensive research has produced fascinating results. It has been observed that patients who haveregular spiritual practices tend to live longer. Self-proclaimed spiritual patients often find strength in theirbeliefs, enabling them better cope with illness, pain, and stress. This inner strength appears to supportpatients enough that their spiritual association is paralleled to enhanced recovery. The power of positivity is strongly tied to a patient's spiritual nature and overall health outcomes are seen in these patients. Practitioners should be familiar with their

Table 1
FICA spiritual history tool©

The acronym FICA can help to structure questions for healthcare professionals who are taking a spiritual history.

F–Faith, Belief, Meaning
"Do you consider yourself to be spiritual?" or "Is spiritually something important to you?"
"Do you have spiritual beliefs, practices, or values that help you to cope with stress, difficult times, or what you are going thorough right now?" (contextualize to visit)
"What gives your life meaning?"

I–Importance and Influence
"What importance does spiritually have in your life?"
"Has your spiritually influenced how you take care of yourself, particularly regarding your health?"
"Does your spiritually affect your healthcare decision making?"

C–Community
"Are you part of a spiritual community?"
"Is your community of support to you and how?" For people who don't identify with a community consider asking "Is there a group of people you really love or who are important to you?" *(Communities such as churches, temples, mosques, family, groups of like-minded friends, or yoga or similar groups can serve as strong support systems for some patients.)*

A–Address/Action in Care
"How would you like me, as your healthcare provider, to address spiritual issues in your healthcare?" *(With newer models, including the diagnosis of spiritual distress, "A" also refers to the "Assessment and Plan" for patient spiritual distress, needs and or resources within a treatment or care plan.)*

© Copyright Christina Puchalski, MD, and The George Washington University 1996 (updated 2022). All rights reserved. Adapted from: Puchalski, C., & Romer, A. L. (2000). Taking a spiritual history allows clinicians to understand patients more fully. Journal of palliative medicine, 3(1), 129-137. Validation study: Tami Borneman, Betty Ferrell, Christina M. Puchalski, Evaluation of the FICA Tool for Spiritual Assessment, Journal of Pain and Symptom Management, 40 (2), 2010, 163-173. https://doi.org/10.1016/j.jpainsymman.2009.12.019.

patient's spiritual beliefs and needs in both an ethicaland medical sense. Jehovah's Witness patients are the classic example. Due to their spiritual values and beliefs, they choose to reject blood transfusions or products. In the clinical arena for instance, when discussing surgical intervention, blood loss is always a risk, and the consenting member of the surgical team must relay that information to the patient as part of their ethical duty of informed consent. The language in this communication is key and proactively recognizing the importance of the patient's spiritual values and the respect to implement their medical decisions without judgement can directly influence the emotion of the interaction and the feelings the patient is left with after the encounter.

There are suggested ethical guidelines for medical professional to incorporate a patient's spiritual care in a respectful and compassionate way. **Practice compassionate presence** – Be fully present and attentive to patients and support them in all of their suffering; physical, emotional, and spiritual. **Listen to patient's fears, hopes, pain, and dreams. Obtain a spiritual history. Be attentive to all dimensions of patients and their families;** body, mind, and spirit. **Incorporate spiritual practices as appropriate. Involve chaplains as members of the disciplinary health care team.**

While the comprehensive idea is a great one, these suggestions can and should be appropriately tailored to the setting where patient care is provided. Per the first line of the Physician Associate Professional Oath, PA's pledge to, "hold as my primary responsibility the health, safety, welfare and dignity of all human beings". 10. While spirituality is not stated verbatim, it is a comprehensive way to incorporate the first point of the oath. Personal and professional boundaries do need to be recognized. Incorporating spirituality may be a delicate balance of actively broaching the subject and passively listening, allowing the patient to guide and lead. It is crucial there are no criticisms or judgements to the patient's response during a spiritual discussion.

Spiritualty has been recognized as a key factor in healthcare. It's a broad concept that may affect not only end-of-life care, but every aspect of patient healthcare. There are many advantages to becoming familiar with a patient's spiritual desires and needs. Incorporating a spiritual history directly aligns with the PA Oath and the FICA method offers easy implementation.

CHALLENGES, ETHICAL DILEMMAS, AND OPPORTUNITIES IN PATIENT EDUCATION

While challenges are plentiful in the medical area, political influence and legal policy has a direct influence on both patients and providers. Just 1 year after a landmark legal case, *Roe v Wade* has been reversed, the obstacles and ethical dilemmas providers face has become exponentially difficult. Fear has been a looming sensation among many practicing in this sensitive arena.[12]

Clinicians have an ethical obligation to practice to the full extent of the law when patient risk requires it, but legal changes have infused endless uncertainty. It is fueled by ambiguous language that demands scrutiny of the exact verbiage. Practitioners are also ethically responsible to take every opportunity to provide personalized medicine discussions and patient education for patients. In the legal sense, the ethical responsibilities provide a blurry outlook. While providers may be fearful of risk of prosecution as an accomplice to a crime to any reinstated law-breaking activity, many simple questions remain unanswered: Is patient counseling toeing the line of breaking the law? Would presenting a patient with a simple decision aid or initiating a comprehensive discussion of their options be viewed as a crime for information sharing? These questions are a few of many that expose the obstacles of the law and leave most feeling that they are widely open to interpretation.

Attempting to dissect this labyrinth leaves a heavy burden. In searching for answers, the preamble to the AMA Code of Ethics states, "When physicians believe a law violates ethical values or is unjust...ethical responsibilities should supersede legal duties."[9] The AMA Code directly acknowledges the enigma, provides guidance with clarity, but another question arises: Are PAs legally protected to follow the AMA oath with the literal verbiage stating "physician"? PAs do have another resource in the PA Code of Ethics beginning with, "Physician Assistants hold as their primary responsibility the health, safety, welfare, and the dignity of all human beings. Physician Assistants uphold the tenets of patient autonomy, beneficence, nonmaleficence, and justice."[10] While this ethical code is clearly denoted for PAs, it sidesteps precise confrontation with the law.

Practice, hospital, and system policies are formulated by ethical and legal team counsels and may also be used as a guide. To examine the baseline foundation for policy decision-making, one should ask what underlying motives the team has. If medical professionals are not included in the writing, a lack of medical expertise and outcome implications may not be considered or weighed heavily. In drawing a parallel to clinicians, legal counsel members must provide advice, or education, based on the most accurate information obtained, and ultimately, the avoidance of corporate risk is at the forefront of these considerations. With a broad analysis of ethical policy creation, it may strengthen or weaken one's confidence in making these unavoidable decisions.

LANGUAGE AND COMMUNICATION

Experts who have studied language barriers find that when individuals experience their nonnative language, they tend to feel foreign language anxiety. Some note that "it is manifest in communication avoidance and withdrawal, as well as code-switching." Results of their investigation find that such communicative behaviors can have a "considerable impact on interpersonal communication, affecting both the content and relationship dimension."[13]

While PAs strive to effectively communicate with their patients and deliver information, when experiencing challenges, they should consider turning to technological advances and innovations. Very frequently in the current landscape of clinical medicine, practitioners are busy, very busy. When thoroughly educating patients by discussing treatment algorithms along with the risks and benefits of each option, patients understandably become lost in the sea of information. Clinical schedules and some diagnoses do not allow for any delay in medical decision-making. Utilizing technology, even in a simple way, may increase patient competence in dealing with information and increase their level of comfort with providers, improving their interactions.[14] The increased use of technology and resources can lead to improved patient outcomes, particularly if they are socially connected for support. In chronic disease processes and health promotion, a literature review supports computer-based patient education having great potential to join and strengthen the classic, robust patient education opportunities.[15]

DECISION AIDS

The value of the patient–provider relationship is limitless, and despite real-world challenges, it can still be well formed, particularly if decision aids are utilized. Decision aids are defined as interventions designed to help people make specific deliberative choices among options by providing information on the options and outcomes relevant to a patient's health. A meta-analysis examining knowledge scores, decisional conflict scores, active patient participation during decision-making, anxiety, and satisfaction found decision aids improve knowledge, reduce decisional conflict, and stimulate patients to be more active in decision-making without increasing their anxiety.[16] If providers create or utilize resources and decision aids, their patients will be better informed and more adept to make clear decisions about their personal values.[17] The challenge will likely be to recognize, then remove personal bias when decision aids are synthesized and ensure that there is a clear delineation between outcomes promoting not just quantity of life, but quality of life as well.[18]

PERSONALIZED MEDICINE

Personalized medicine, also recognized as precision medicine, describes the tailoring of patient treatment to individual patients. To zoom in on the widely recognized genetics field of study, this describes pharmacogenomics. In clinical application, providers take a pharmacogenomic report, an analysis of how the genetic makeup of a patient affects their response to drugs and prescribes pharmacotherapy with purpose and intention. While this is an exciting and promising field, prescribers should not lose sight of the complete patient in front of them. Just as patients are more than any of their data, they are also more than their genetic structure. In widening our lens, clinicians who utilize pharmacogenomics are gifted the opportunity to individualize pharmacotherapy, but all medical decisions, practices, and interventions may be personalized to a patient to some degree. The definitions of personalized medicine ironically focus on standardized algorithms and exclude any personal interaction with the patient being treated.

It is hardly a novel idea that active decisions instead of passive are necessary when taking care of patients. It is easy to become swept away by the newer practices in medicine, which focus on standardizations, coding, and algorithms not frequently formulated by licensed medical providers. Formal guidelines are a rigid system, typically reliant upon International Classification of Diseases (ICD) coding, which indicate a one-size-fits-most approach. These guidelines are often viewed as nonmalleable, but the beauty of personalized medicine in an educational sense includes patient preference and sometimes the best plan may stray from this worn path of processes. It is apparent that in order to incorporate patient preference, thorough patient education must be provided to ensure quality shared decision-making.[18]

THE FUTURE OF PATIENT EDUCATION IN THE TWENTY-FIRST CENTURY

In terms of ethical considerations and the future directions in patient education, emerging technologies and innovations, particularly artificial intelligence (AI), Change is constant and with the newer models of patient education, relationship building is the cornerstone of excellent patient care.[3,8] Without speaking the same language, effective communication, particularly when discussing the details of one's major health decisions, is lost. In the United States' diversified population, the need for multilingual communication is exploding. Since the 1950s, machine translation, or automated translation, has been common but has severe limitations in accuracy. In a high-stakes medical discussion, practitioners cannot tolerate validity being a concern, particularly when the awareness of litigation can quickly loom nearby. Perfection is rarely expected, but what is unintentionally lost in translation could swiftly lead to patient harm. Legal implications are a concrete consequence, but when faced with realistic challenges of urgent need and lack of alternatives, is there a best route?[19] Providers need to consider that while there have been vast advancements, given when deciding to use a translation tool, careful consideration should be not replacing professional verbal communication when discussing sensitive medical subject matter.[20]

The future of patient education has scope for growth and should be a collaboration of emerging technology with classic provider involvement. AI has become the hot topic for innovation in nearly every field. Radiology has been touted as the gateway for AI implementation into the medical realm. By definition, AI is a composition of devices or systems that can perceive some element of their environment and use this information to achieve a predefined goal.[21] In the field of radiology, AI has been utilized for scheduling and protocoling as well as optimizing workflow. The American College of Radiology gives implementation outcomes such as reduced wait times, improved communication with patients, and even tailored examinations that are reminiscent of a personalized medicine approach in radiology. With progression, AI is being trialed with image interpretation and intelligent reporting systems. The opportunities seem limitless, and AI implementation in health care seems no different. Despite its challenges, many find it appealing with a major advantage of reducing overall health care costs. Looking forward, other data endpoints should be examined to establish a true outcome measurement if implementation is successful into daily practice. The major red flag on being too reliant on any technology is the lack of human oversight. With only data, and without empathy and emotion, there are several ethical concerns with utilizing AI as an accepted standard of care method for medical decision-making. Finding the delicate balance of data output analysis, personalized medicine approaches, and health care goals proves to be a difficult task.

One recent battle regarding AI is aimed toward insurance companies. Class action suits have been filed against these conglomerates with accusations of utilizing AI to systematically deny necessary care placements and treatments. The cornerstone of the issue is the AI model functions by supplying data-driven output after analyzing database input. In trying to emulate the efficiency and cost-savings the radiology sector has found major obstacles have been encountered and the issue came to a head. The legal result is a 2 fold implementation of new federal laws prohibiting Medicare Advantage plans from "relying on an algorithm or software to make medically necessary determinations" and mandating "any medical necessity denial" to be "reviewed."[22] Further details are lacking with a specific review protocol, but with the vast implementation of AI across the medical field, inevitable legal changes are proving to be reactive than proactive.

DISCLOSURE

The authors have nothing to disclose.

REFERENCES

1. Borza LR, Gavrilovici C, Stockman R. Ethical models of physician-patient relationship revisited with regard to patient autonomy, values, and patient education. The Medical-Surgical Journal 2015;119(2).
2. Emanuel EJ, Emanuel LL. Four models of the physician-patient relationship. JAMA 1992;267(16):2221–6.
3. Berger R, Bulmash B, Dron N, et al. The patient-physician relationship: an account of the physician's perspective. Isr J Health Pol Res 2020;9:33.
4. Chang CS, Chen SY, Lan YT. Service quality, trust, and patient satisfaction in interpersonal-based medical service encounters. BMC Health Serv Res 2013;13(1):1–15.
5. Inui TS, Carter WB, Kukull WA, et al. Outcome-based doctor-patient interaction analysis: comparison of techniques. Med Care 1982;20(6):535–49.
6. Redman BK. Ethics of patient education and how do we make it everyone's ethics. Nurs Clin North Am 2011;46(3):283–9.
7. Redman BK. When is patient education unethical? Nurs Ethics 2008;15:813–20.
8. Agarwal AK, Murinson BB. New dimensions in patient-physician interaction: values, autonomy, and medical information in the patient-centered clinical encounter. Rambam Maimonides Med. J 2012;3(3):e0017.
9. American Medical Association. Code of Ethics. Available at: https://code-medical-ethics.ama-assn.org/principles.
10. American Academy of Physician Associates. Code of Ethics. Available at: https://www.aapa.org/career-central/practice-tools/ethical-guidelines-for-the-pa-profession/.
11. Puchalski CM. The role of spirituality in health care. Baylor University Medical Center Proceedings 2001;14(4):352–7.
12. Watson K, Oberman M. Abortion counseling, liability, and the first amendment. N Engl J Med 2023;389(7):663–7.
13. Aichorn N, Puck J. "I just don't feel comfortable speaking English": foreign language anxiety as a catalyst for spoken-language barriers in MNCs. Int Bus Rev 2017;26(4):749–63.

14. Gustafson DH, Hawkins R, Pingree S, et al. Effect of computer support on younger women with breast cancer. J Gen Intern Med 2001;16(7):435–45.

15. Lewis D. Computer-based approaches to patient education: A review of the literature. J Am Med Inf Assoc 1999;6(4):272–82.

16. O'Connor AM, Rostom A, Fiset V, et al. Decision aids for patients facing health treatment or screening decisions: Systematic review. BMJ 1999;319(7212): 731–4.

17. Stacey D, Légaré F, Lewis K, et al. Decision aids for people facing health treatment or screening decisions. Cochrane Database Syst Rev 2017;4. https://doi.org/10.1002/14651858.cd001431.pub5.

18. Van Weert JC, van Munster BC, Sanders R, et al. Decision aids to help older people make health decisions: A systematic review and meta-analysis. BMC Med Inf Decis Making 2016;16(1).

19. Vieira LN, O'Hagan M, O'Sullivan C. Understanding the societal impacts of machine translation: A critical review of the literature on medical and legal use cases. Inf Commun Soc 2020;1–18.

20. Panayiotou A, Gardner A, Williams S, et al. Language translation apps in health care settings: expert opinion. JMIR mHealth and uHealth 2019;7(4). https://doi.org/10.2196/11316.

21. Zoga A, Ali S. Artificial intelligence in radiology: current technology and future directions. Semin Muscoskel Radiol 2018;22(5):540–5.

22. Weber S. UHC accused of using AI to Skirt doctors' orders, deny claims. Medscape Business of Medicine 2023.

Leveraging Advanced Physician Assistant/Associate Credentials for Patient Education

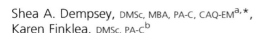

Shea A. Dempsey, DMSc, MBA, PA-C, CAQ-EM[a],[*],
Karen Finklea, DMSc, PA-C[b]

KEYWORDS

- Physician Assistant/Associate • Doctorate • Residency • Fellowship
- Certificate of added qualifications • Credentials • Patient education

KEY POINTS

- Advanced credentials for physician assistants/associates (PAs) can aid in fostering advanced clinical competence and may contribute to empowering evidence-based patient education.
- Certificates of Added Qualifications provide customized education based on specialty that can help address patient needs.
- Accessibility and finances are barriers to leveraging advanced PA credentials; however, some regulatory considerations and processes should be advocated.
- PAs have 4 national governing organizations that work to future-proof credentialing and licensing practices and maintain health care practices above standards.

INTRODUCTION

Advances in medical education have led to many efficiencies within the health care field. Health care providers have an overarching medical goal to provide safe, compassionate care to all. A significant component of providing care is ensuring patient education. There is an innate need for health care literacy among all individuals. As of 2022, individuals aged 65 years or older in the United States represent 17.3% (~55 million) of the population.[1] Simply put, people are living longer as scientific developments and modern medicine evolve. However, health literacy among patients and those on a health care team is needed to continue this effort of lengthy livelihood.

[a] Shenandoah University, 1775 N Sector Court, Suite 200, Winchester, VA 22601, USA; [b] 82 Holland Street, Rochester, NY 14605, USA
* Corresponding author.
E-mail address: sdempsey09@su.edu

Physician Assist Clin 9 (2024) 655–664
https://doi.org/10.1016/j.cpha.2024.05.014
physicianassistant.theclinics.com
2405-7991/24/© 2024 Elsevier Inc. All rights are reserved, including those for text and data mining, AI training, and similar technologies.

Physician assistants/associates (PAs) have a dynamic role in caring for patients while playing a crucial part in providing exemplary patient education.

The PA profession was initially created in the 1960s as a buffer to aid in the shortage of primary care physicians. Navy corpsmen were trained in generalized medicine initially at Duke University to serve alongside physicians and help with the demand and need.[2] Particularly, rural communities were concerned about the lack of health care promoted in these areas. Before long, PAs were an integral part of the health care team setting. Since then, the PA profession has expanded academically and career-wise in various ways.

PAs are lifelong learners who continuously advance their knowledge of medicine within their respective specialties. This learning occurs through independent learning, research, preceptorship, or continuing medical education certifications.

With the expansion of the roles of PAs within health care, additional opportunities are available to provide PAs with the learning opportunity promoting health literacy to their patients. Residency programs and Certificates of Added Qualifications (CAQs) were created for PAs who wanted to advance their evidence-based medical knowledge in specialty care. In addition, the first publicly available clinical doctoral degree program available for PAs was created at Nova Southeastern University in Florida.[3] All these have played a role in preparing PAs to provide their patients with the best evidence-based education and care.

This article aims to delve deeper into each educational opportunity afforded to advance PA credentials. Each opportunity further equips PAs with health literacy for efficient patient care while providing credence to advance the PA profession.

EMPOWERING PATIENT EDUCATION THROUGH DOCTORAL DEGREES

One way PAs can elevate their practice and expand their ability to provide quality patient education is to pursue advanced education through a doctoral degree. While PAs can pursue any number of advanced degrees, 2 of the most prominent options include the Doctor of Medical Science (DMS(c)) and the Doctor of Health Science (DHSc), followed by PhD, EdD, and MD.[4]

The DMS(c) degree is an advanced, clinical doctorate designed for PAs seeking to enhance their clinical expertise, leadership skills, and research capabilities.[5] The DMS(c) degree equips graduates with the expertise to critically appraise and apply research findings, contribute to the advancement of clinical practice, and potentially pursue academic or leadership roles within health care. All programs offering a DMS(c) degree require students to be a physician assistant with the exception of 1 program; Northeastern University is open to any health care professional with a bachelor's degree or master's degree.[6] While individual program and curricular design may vary from one institution to another, the degree is offered to physician assistants and may help open doors to career advancement in leadership, education, research, and even commercial industry careers.

The (DHSc) degree builds upon previous health professional degrees and while (DHSc) may offer similar content as the DMS(c), this degree is open to all health professionals. While the first DMS(c) degree was not offered until 2016 at Lincoln Memorial University,[7] the DHS(c) had been available since 1999, first offered at the University of St. Augustine for Health Sciences.[8] Baylor University offered a residency in emergency medicine that culminated with earning the Doctor of Science in Physician Assistant Studies, DScPAS-EM, although this program was limited to military PAs, and not publicly available to civilian PAs.[9] Given that there were no publicly available PA-specific doctoral degrees until recently, many PAs pursued the DMS(c) that provided advanced education on health policy, public health, leadership, medical education, and research.

New PAs graduate with a master's degree; however, this was not always the case. PAs have entered the workforce with certificate training, associate degrees, bachelor's degrees, and master's degrees. While some medical knowledge never changes, like the number of bones in the body, the demands of patients and employers are larger than ever before. This necessitates that PAs be equipped to successfully manage patients and the health care system in the 21st century. Interestingly, all these PAs with varying degrees all take the same board examination and obtain the same certification by the National Certification Commission of Physician Assistants. There is no additional board examination, licensure, or certification that any PA gets by completing a doctoral degree, but yet there is still value. While all PAs take the same initial board examination, PAs pursuing their CAQ will take additional examinations as part of their CAQ process.

PAs with doctoral degrees often pursue these options as they may have interest in leadership, research, or education. These skills of understanding scholarly work and educating others could translate into improved patient education as well. Doctorally prepared PAs are required to assess current literature and stay abreast of medical advances and changes. This means that these PAs have additional training in interpreting and sharing current research as it applies to their patients, including patient education.

The big question is WHY? Why does it make a difference? The word doctor stems from the Latin word meaning teacher.[10] Once someone has the training of doctoral education, they are to have mastered the information, understand how to access new information, and teach that information to others. While being an effective teacher is not limited to those with doctoral education, having a doctoral degree does provide evidence of the training completed. Patients benefit as patients are more likely to participate in their medical care and medical outcomes improve when patients have a better understanding of their medical diagnosis and treatment plan.[11] This means patients do better when they understand the "WHY." Who better to educate patients than the doctorally prepared PA clinician caring for the patient? Doctoral education has the potential to enhance competency in patient education.

Specialization and Expertise: The Certificate of Added Qualification Advantage

The National Commission on Certification of Physician Assistants (NCCPA) board of directors approved a motion to implement CAQs in 2009.[12] The idea behind CAQs in the PA profession was to create a dynamic approach in which individuals had the opportunity to show their extended knowledge and care base within a given field.[4] NCCPA administered the first CAQ in September 2011.[12] Since its implementation, more than 2400 PAs have taken a CAQ within their designated specialty.[13] The overall number of PAs eligible for a CAQ within their specialty remains low for several reasons. However, PAs who have obtained a CAQ have noted significant benefits. In addition to showing an in-depth knowledge of a given specialty, PAs who have a CAQ endorsed additional accolades of success promotion, increase in job responsibilities, pay increases, cash bonuses, and greater respect and acceptance from patients.[12]

Approved PA CAQ examinations have grown in number since their inception. To date, there are 8 approved CAQs by NCCPA (**Box 1**).[13]

Unsurprisingly, the CAQ in emergency medicine is held by more PAs than any other CAQ, and psychiatry has the highest percentage of PAs practicing in a specialty who hold the CAQ.[13] Each CAQ specialty showcases medical competency in a specified PA specialty. The CAQ requires extensive preparation to succeed in passing. It allows

---

Box 1
Current approved physician assistant/associate certificates of added qualifications by the National Commission on Certification of Physician Assistants

Approved CAQs by NCCPA
  Cardiovascular and Thoracic Surgery
  Dermatology
  Emergency Medicine
  Hospital Medicine
  Nephrology
  Palliative Medicine and Hospice Care
  Pediatrics
  Psychiatry
  Obstetrics and Gynecology
  Occupational Medicine
  Orthopedic Surgery

PAs to reflect as they can look back on missed information. As a result, PAs can change their way of practicing medicine to treat their patients' needs using evidence-based concepts appropriately. Essential prerequisites for PAs to be approved to take the CAQ: having a current Physician Assistant - Certified (PA-C) certification, an unrestricted PA license, a minimum of 75 credits of Category I CME, and 4000 clinical hours or experience.[12] The minimum requirements were approved to show clinical experience and knowledge within the specialty.

The CAQ examination provides PAs with the opportunity to reflect. PAs can study standard disease processes in their specialty and continuously update their thought process on treating patients. As a result, patients are being treated with updated medical care. Research on patient education and satisfaction with PAs who have a CAQ and its correlation to overall patient health literacy is limited; however, there has been some research within physician CAQ examinations and nursing specialty certifications to demonstrate a positive connection. Clinical reviews throughout the years show no overall clinical significance in patient satisfaction when care is provided by a PA versus physician versus nurse practitioner.[14] Research showed the benefits of skilled nursing staff who obtained specialty certification. Similar to the PA CAQ examinations, clinical prerequisites have been established for nurses seeking additional certifications within their specialty. Competency and passing of these certifications resulted in a link between self-validation and personal satisfaction secondary to improved quality care and patient outcomes.[15] Although further research is warranted, as nursing certifications, CAQs for PAs will hopefully show positive contributions to addressing the needs of patients.

Clinical Excellence and Patient-Centric Residency Programs

When PAs graduate from PA school, they all take the same board examination and technically can be hired into any specialty. The education in the PA program cannot prepare students for every scenario in every specialty but rather focuses on the building blocks needed by the majority of PAs, typically with a focus on primary care and the curriculum for PA schools must meet accreditation standards by the Accreditation Review Commission on Education for the Physician Assistant (ARC-PA).[16,17] While recently the ARC-PA has started to reaccredit postgraduate education like residencies and fellowships, only 5.4% of all PAs have completed postgraduate training like a residency or fellowship.[4,16] So what does the residency offer?

Most PA residency or fellowships last between 12 and 18 months and offer focused curriculum in specific medical disciplines such as pediatric surgery, critical care, emergency medicine, orthopedics, transplant surgery, and rural medicine.[9] When attending a residency or fellowship, the PA will choose 1 with a specific discipline; however, that will not be the only discipline taught during the residency. Both PA residents and fellows will have both didactic and practical education, off service appointments in other disciplines in an effort to understand how other disciplines may impact their own service, as the entire time that they are learning, they have supervision and guidance to practice and hone their skills.[17] The entire time that residents and fellows are completing their training, they are practicing PAs with a license to practice medicine. This means that they are seeing patients, creating treatment plans, diagnosing, educating patients, making referrals, and all the while getting guided support, feedback, and critique to improve all these skills.

How does this additional training in a residency or fellowship impact patient education? Physician assistant providers have a very accelerated or condensed learning curve when completing a residency or fellowship, and when complete, typically have the knowledge, skillset, and experience that would have taken several years to obtain otherwise.[18] As providers gain experience, they have more to guide their future experiences. They have learned from mistakes in a supervised environment and now have the opportunity to be exposed to a large number of patients within their medical discipline and beyond. This experience guides compassion, empathy, and the PA fellow has had didactic and practical experience to guide patient discussions with knowledge appropriate for the encounter.[17]

OVERCOMING CHALLENGES AND ENSURING PATIENT-CENTERED CARE

As earlier discussed, only about 5.4% of PAs have attended any postgraduate medical training like a residency or fellowship.[4] So why are not more PA providers attending postgraduate training? The answers may not be as straightforward as desired; however, there are many factors to consider. Some PAs may have a desire to work in primary care, or another specialty that does not have a residency. Others may not be in the situation in life to take a financial hit. Most PA postgraduate programs pay $40,000–$75,000 annually, which is much lower than typical PA jobs; all the while many PAs likely just graduated with a mountain of student loans, the average being $115,000 in debt.[17,19] When considering starting a career, the PA must weigh the benefits of attending a postgraduate residency against the costs of taking a lower salary, interest adding up on student loans, and possibly another year before they could be in the position or geographic location they want to be.

There are definite opportunities to improve access to postgraduate PA residencies and fellowships, and the first would include incentivized funding to the organization as well as the PA. Physician medical residencies are federally funded; however, there are no specific federal funding for PA postgraduate programs, even though there are over 140,000 practicing PAs caring for patients in the United States.[20] Second, since PA residents are licensed PAs, they are billing for services rendered during their training. Regardless of training or experience, Medicare and other insurances only reimburse at 85% of the agreed upon rate when compared to physician colleagues for the same service.[21] This lesser reimbursement implies that the patient received subpar care yet could not be further from the truth. Physician assistants often increase access to care and decrease wait times, which patients appreciate and improves patient education.[22] Changing reimbursement to outcomes based, rather than a percentage of fee-for-service, could increase revenue available to PAs and postgraduate residency programs.

As more postgraduate residences become available, they start to look a little more similar and streamlined. Accreditation standards also help to standardize the required curriculum, patient exposures, competencies, and outcomes. Although ARC-PA has started to offer voluntary accreditation of postgraduate residencies and fellowships, there is nothing in their competencies or clinical postgraduate standards that address patient education as a competency or skill.[23] This does not mean that programs are not emphasizing this, but rather it is not required by accreditation, and therefore, the quality of this skill may not be standardized from one program to another or demonstrate proficiency. When PAs are able to practice a skill such as patient education in a structured postgraduate residency or fellowship, they can sharpen these skills and take them to positively impact patient education for the remainder of their career.

Currently, accreditation for postgraduate PA residencies and fellowships is voluntary and ARC-PA is one of the accrediting bodies offering accreditation; however, there are other organizations that programs can seek accreditation.[23,24] Given that accreditation is voluntary and there are several organizations that can provide this review, the standardization and quality of education from one program to another cannot be validated. Completing a post graduate residency or fellowship does not change or affect national certification or licensure currently. However, state legislation is constantly changing, so licensure requirements and scope of practice are subject to change. Some specialties offer CAQs, which have a standardized examination and attestation of skills and hours worked in a specialty. Completing a postgraduate residency or fellowship could accelerate the PA toward a CAQ.[12] As time continues, there will be a regression toward the mean with postgraduate residencies and fellowships which will make the process and standards much more streamlined. Although in the meantime, standardizing accreditation as well as pathways toward CAQ will help to simplify the process and increase the value of the training.

ANTICIPATING FUTURE TRENDS AND INNOVATIONS

As health care education evolves, the PA profession needs an equitable educational background like other disciplines. The accepted terminal degree of certified PAs is a master's level education with a didactic classroom experience and clinical averaging 27 months.

As the PA role has expanded over the decades, we now see the profession's expansion in other health care-related fields: education, administration, leadership, and research. Consideration has been applied to whether the PA profession should boost their terminal degree to the doctorate level. Formal arrangements have yet to be made to accept the doctoral degree as terminal. Continuous thought is given to PA certification and acknowledging minimum academic education.

The PA profession has accrediting and credentialing practices that are supported by 4 independent organizations: the American Academy of Physician Associates (AAPA), the ARC-PA, the NCCPA, and the PA Education Association. Each organization continues to uphold the standards set forth to promote the integrity of the PA profession.

Founded in 1968, AAPA serves as the national governing body within the United States to support and advance the PA profession and provide awareness to the public.[2] NCCPA was founded in 1974 as the certification body for PAs in the United States.[25] NCCPA serves to test the clinical acumen of practicing PAs. New graduate PAs meeting class requirements can sit for the Physician Assistant National Certifying

Exam. Upon passing this examination, the PAs are certified to obtain licensure in any of the 50 states. A 2 year maintenance certification is required as a means that fosters lifelong learning. PAs must report at least 100 hours of certified medical education every 2 years as practicing PAs. PAs prove their clinical knowledge every 10 years through the Physician Assistant National Recertifying Exam.

The Physician Assistant Education Association (PAEA) was founded in 1972 under the Association of Physician Assistant Programs.[26] The PAEA serves as the governing body for PA education, with all accredited programs within the United States participating. The PAEA provides updated resources and support to PA faculty and individuals interested in providing PA education.

Similar to the PAEA, the ARC-PA supports PA education. ARC-PA was developed in 1971 under the American Medical Association.[27] After several decades of collaboration, ARC-PA became a standalone accrediting body for the PA programs, which has included accreditation protocol for clinical postgraduate PA programs.[27] ARC-PA maintains a standard of reviewing each program is maintaining standards that are patient-centered by having PA program renew their accreditation every 10 years, sometimes sooner depending on circumstances.

Advocacy of the PA profession is imperative in bringing awareness to the public about how we contribute and provide patient-centered care. Each of these organizations joins forces in future-proofing the credentialing and licensing practices of PAs.

SUMMARY: FORGING THE PATH TO ENHANCED PATIENT EDUCATION

This article highlighting advanced credentials for PAs outlines the evolving landscape for PAs and their pivotal role in patient education. It underscores how educational advancements, including doctoral degrees, CAQs, and postgraduate training, enhance PA practice and benefit patient education. The growing number of PAs seeking advanced degrees like the DMS(c) and DHSc highlights the commitment of PAs to continuous learning and expertise expansion. These programs empower PAs to engage in leadership, research, and education, fostering a deeper understanding of medical knowledge and the ability to translate it effectively to patients.

The discussion on CAQs further exemplifies the dedication of PAs toward specialized knowledge, showcasing competency in various specialties. While not mandatory, obtaining a CAQ brings benefits like professional recognition, career advancement, and trusted evaluated standard when educating patients.

Additionally, the significance of postgraduate training, like residencies and fellowships, becomes evident. These programs offer focused education, allowing PAs to refine their skills, gain diverse experiences, and ultimately enhance patient education by providing more comprehensive and informed care.

Despite the merits, challenges in accessing postgraduate programs exist, including financial considerations and lack of standardized competencies addressing patient education.. Addressing these hurdles could encourage more PAs to pursue further training, benefiting both their professional growth and patient care.

This underscores the value of postgraduate credentials, and the benefits patients receive including improved patient education. However, there is still a need for continued evolution in, improving access to training, and clear communication to the public regarding the value of advanced PA credentials. Collaboration among organizations representing the PA profession, certification, and training remains crucial in shaping a future where skilled and knowledgeable PAs contribute to optimal patient care through enhanced health care literacy and patient education.

CLINICS CARE POINTS

- Doctoral Degrees and Patient Education:
  - Doctoral degrees like the DMS(c) and DHSc enhance PAs' clinical expertise, leadership, and research skills, contributing to improved patient education.
- Doctoral education prepares PAs to critically appraise and apply research findings to patient education and care. Certificates of Added Qualifications (CAQs):
  - CAQs demonstrate the PA's knowledge and skill in a specific medical field, and require ongoing education to maintain.
- Obtaining a CAQ can lead to professional recognition, career advancement, and improved patient trust and satisfaction. Postgraduate Residency and Fellowship Programs:
  - Residency and fellowship programs offer intensive, focused training in specific medical disciplines, accelerating the PA's learning curve and expertise.
- These programs include both didactic and practical education, allowing PAs to refine their skills, which can directly benefit patient care and patient education. Health Literacy and Patient Education:
  - Effective patient education is linked to improved health outcomes and patient participation in their care.
  - PAs with advanced credentials have additional experience and skillset to provide patients with excellent education.

DISCLOSURE

The authors declare no financial gains or conflicts of interest related to the information presented in this article.

REFERENCES

1. Explore Census Data. data.census.gov. Available at: https://data.census.gov/profile/United_States?g=010XX00US. [Accessed 15 October 2023].
2. AAPA. History of the PA Profession and the American Academy of PAs - AAPA. AAPA 2016. Available at: https://www.aapa.org/about/history/. [Accessed 28 October 2023].
3. MILESTONES in PA HISTORY. Available at: https://www.aapa.org/wp-content/uploads/2017/01/History_Milestones.pdf. [Accessed 29 November 2023].
4. National Commission on Certification of Physician Assistants. 2022 statistical profile of certified physician assistants [annual report]. 2023. Available at: https://www.nccpa.net/wp-content/uploads/2023/04/2022-Statistical-Profile-of-Board-Certified-PAs.pdf. [Accessed 2 November 2023].
5. Miller AA, Coplan B. Assessing the economics of an entry-level physician assistant doctoral degree. J Physician Assist Educ 2022;33(1):34–40.
6. Northeastern University. Healthcare leadership: doctor of medical science in healthcare leadership. 2023. Available at: https://graduate.northeastern.edu/program/doctor-of-medical-science-in-healthcare-leadership-19118/. [Accessed 3 November 2023].
7. Lincoln Memorial University. Doctor of Medical Science Program. Available at: https://www.lmunet.edu/school-of-medical-sciences/dms/index#:~:text=The%20clinical%20medicine%20major%20was,medical%20training%20to%20Physician%20Assistants. [Accessed 3 November 2023].
8. University of St. Augustine for Health Sciences. Our history. Available at: https://www.usa.edu/about/history-of-university-of-st-augustine-for-health-sciences/. [Accessed 3 November 2023].

9. Emergency Medicine, DSc.P.A. < Baylor University. catalog.baylor.edu. Available at: https://catalog.baylor.edu/grauate-school/affiliated-programs/physician-assistant/emergency-medcine-dscpa/. [Accessed 17 April 2024].

10. Merriam-Webster. The history of 'Doctor'. Available at: https://www.merriam-webster.com/wordplay/the-history-of-doctor. [Accessed 18 November 2023].

11. Paterick TE, Patel N, Tajik AJ, et al. Improving Health Outcomes Through Patient Education and Partnerships with Patients. Proc (Bayl Univ Med Cent) 2017;30(1): 112–3.

12. National Commission on Certification of Physician Assistants. Certificates of Added Qualifications. Available at: https://www.nccpa.net/specialty-certificates/. [Accessed 8 November 2023].

13. National Commission of Certification of Physician Assistants. 2021 statistical profile of board certified PAs by state. 2023. Available at: https://www.nccpa.net/wp-content/uploads/2023/02/2021-State-Report-2_13_23.pdf. [Accessed 13 November 2023].

14. Hooker RS, Moloney-Johns AJ, McFarland MM. Patient satisfaction with physician assistant/associate care: an international scoping review. Hum Resour Health 2019;17(1). https://doi.org/10.1186/s12960-019-0428-7.

15. Whitehead L, Ghosh M, Walker DK, et al. The relationship between specialty nurse certification and patient, nurse and organizational outcomes: A systematic review. Int J Nurs Stud 2019;93:1–11.

16. Accreditation Review Commission on education for the Physician Assistant. About ARC-PA. Available at: https://www.arc-pa.org/about/. [Accessed 4 November 2023].

17. American Association of Surgical Physician Assistants. PA Residency Programs. Available at: https://www.aaspa.com/pa-residency-programs. [Accessed 7 November 2023].

18. The Association of Post Graduate PA Programs. Advantages of Post Graduate Residency and Fellowship Programs. Available at: https://appap.mypanetwork.com/page/1208-advantages-of-postgraduate-residency-and-fellowship-programs. [Accessed 6 November 2023].

19. Baker A. PA Student Financial Decision Making:What you need to know. PA Foundation. 2022. Available at: https://pa-foundation.org/in-the-words-of-pas/pa-student-financial-decision-making-what-you-need-to-know/. [Accessed 6 November 2023].

20. United States Bureau of Labor Statistics. Occupational Employment and Wages May 2022; Physician Assistant. Available at: https://www.bls.gov/oes/current/oes291071.htm. [Accessed 5 November 2023].

21. American Academy of Physician Associates. Third Party Reimbursement for PAs. 2018. Available at: https://www.aapa.org/wp-content/uploads/2017/01/Third_party_payment_2017_FINAL.pdf. [Accessed 5 November 2023].

22. Godley M, Jenkins JB. Decreasing wait times and increasing patient satisfaction: a lean six sigma approach. J Nurs Care Qual 2019;34(1):61–5.

23. Accreditation Review Commission on education for the Physician Assistant. Accreditation Review Standards for Clinical Postgraduate PA Programs. Available at: https://www.arc-pa.org/wp-content/uploads/2021/12/Clinical-Postgraduate-Standards-3rd-Edition-with-clarfifications-as-of-October-2021-1.pdf. [Accessed 10 November 2023].

24. Consortium for Advanced Practice Providers. Eligibility for Accreditation Review. Available at: https://www.apppostgradtraining.com/accreditation/eligibility-accreditation-review/. [Accessed 12 November 2023].

25. National Commission on Certification of Physician Assistants. About us. Available at: https://www.nccpa.net/about-nccpa/. [Accessed 14 November 2023].

26. PA Education Association. About us. Available at: https://paeaonline.org/our-work/about-us. [Accessed 30 October 2023].

27. Accreditation Review Commission on Education for the Physician Assistant. Accreditation committee/commission history timeline. Available at: https://www.arc-pa.org/about/arc-pa-history. [Accessed 4 November 2023].

Moving?

Make sure your subscription moves with you!

To notify us of your new address, find your **Clinics Account Number** (located on your mailing label above your name), and contact customer service at:

Email: journalscustomerservice-usa@elsevier.com

800-654-2452 (subscribers in the U.S. & Canada)
314-447-8871 (subscribers outside of the U.S. & Canada)

Fax number: 314-447-8029

Elsevier Health Sciences Division
Subscription Customer Service
3251 Riverport Lane
Maryland Heights, MO 63043

ELSEVIER